THE VALUE OF BCG AND TNF IN AUTOIMMUNITY

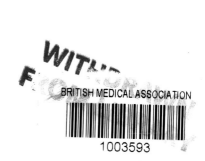

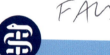

THE VALUE OF BCG AND TNF IN AUTOIMMUNITY

Second Edition

Edited by

DENISE L. FAUSTMAN

Director of Immunobiology, Massachusetts General Hospital,
Boston, MA, United States
Associate Professor of Medicine, Harvard Medical School,
Boston, MA, United States

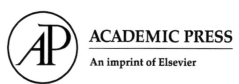

ACADEMIC PRESS

An imprint of Elsevier

Academic Press is an imprint of Elsevier
125 London Wall, London EC2Y 5AS, United Kingdom
525 B Street, Suite 1650, San Diego, CA 92101, United States
50 Hampshire Street, 5th Floor, Cambridge, MA 02139, United States
The Boulevard, Langford Lane, Kidlington, Oxford OX5 1GB, United Kingdom

Notices

Knowledge and best practice in this field are constantly changing. As new research and experience
broaden our understanding, changes in research methods, professional practices, or medical treatment
may become necessary.

Practitioners and researchers must always rely on their own experience and knowledge in evaluating
and using any information, methods, compounds, or experiments described herein. In using such
information or methods they should be mindful of their own safety and the safety of others, including
parties for whom they have a professional responsibility.

To the fullest extent of the law, neither the Publisher nor the authors, contributors, or editors, assume
any liability for any injury and/or damage to persons or property as a matter of products liability,
negligence or otherwise, or from any use or operation of any methods, products, instructions, or ideas
contained in the material herein.

Library of Congress Cataloging-in-Publication Data
A catalog record for this book is available from the Library of Congress

British Library Cataloguing-in-Publication Data
A catalogue record for this book is available from the British Library

ISBN: 978-0-12-814603-3

For information on all Academic Press publications
visit our website at https://www.elsevier.com/books-and-journals

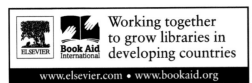

Working together
to grow libraries in
developing countries

www.elsevier.com • www.bookaid.org

Publisher: Mica Haley
Acquisition Editor: Linda Versteeg-Buschman
Editorial Project Manager: Kristi Anderson
Production Project Manager: Punithavathy Govindaradjane
Cover Designer: Miles Hitchen

Typeset by SPi Global, India

DEDICATION

This updated edition of *The Value of BCG and TNF in Autoimmunity* is dedicated to Bob Glenister whose creativity and generosity have been the driving force behind this unique and important global collaboration. Bob, on behalf of the researchers you have inspired and the patients whose lives we hope to improve, thank you.

CONTENTS

4. Host Epigenetic Modifications in *Mycobacterium tuberculosis* Infection: A Boon or Bane   **39**
Mona Singh, Vinod Yadav, Gobardhan Das

5. Mycobacterium Bovis Bacille Calmette-Guerin Vaccination: Can Biomarkers Predict Efficacy?   **57**
Hazel M. Dockrell

6. The Heterologous Effects of Bacillus Calmette-Guérin (BCG) Vaccine and Trained Innate Immunity   **71**
Boris Novakovic, Nicole L. Messina, Nigel Curtis

CONTRIBUTORS

P. Aaby
Research Center for Vitamins and Vaccines (CVIVA), Copenhagen S, Denmark; Bandim Health Project, Indepth Network, Bissau, Guinea-Bissau

Rob J.W. Arts
Department of Internal Medicine and Radboud Center for Infectious Diseases, Radboud University Medical Center, Nijmegen, The Netherlands

C.S. Benn
Research Center for Vitamins and Vaccines (CVIVA), Copenhagen S; OPEN, Institute of Clinical Research and Danish Institute of Advanced Science, University of Southern Denmark and Odense University Hospital, Odense, Denmark

Nina Marie Birk
Department of Paediatrics, Copenhagen University Hospital, Hvidovre, Denmark

Barry R. Bloom
Harvard T.H. Chan School of Public Health, Boston, MA, United States

Natalie Bruiners
Public Health Research Institute, New Jersey Medical School, Rutgers, The State University of New Jersey, Newark, NJ, United States

Maria Chiara Buscarinu
Center for Experimental Neurological Therapies S. Andrea Hospital-site, Neurosciences, Mental Health, and Sensory Organs (NESMOS) Department, "Sapienza" University of Rome, Rome, Italy

Nigel Curtis
Cancer & Disease Epigenetics and Infectious Diseases & Microbiology Research Groups, Murdoch Children's Research Institute; Department of Paediatrics, The University of Melbourne; Infectious Diseases Unit, The Royal Children's Hospital Melbourne, Parkville, VIC, Australia

Gobardhan Das
Special Centre for Molecular Medicine, Jawaharlal Nehru University, New Delhi, India

Hazel M. Dockrell
Department of Immunology and Infection, London School of Hygiene & Tropical Medicine, London, United Kingdom

Denise L. Faustman
Director of Immunobiology, Massachusetts General Hospital; Associate Professor of Medicine, Harvard Medical School, Boston, MA, United States

Michela Ferraldeschi
Department of Neurology and Psychiatry, "Sapienza" University of Rome, Rome, Italy

Arianna Fornasiero
Center for Experimental Neurological Therapies S. Andrea Hospital-site, Neurosciences, Mental Health, and Sensory Organs (NESMOS) Department, "Sapienza" University of Rome, Rome, Italy

Maria Laura Gennaro
Public Health Research Institute, New Jersey Medical School, Rutgers, The State University of New Jersey, Newark, NJ, United States

Valentina Guerrini
Public Health Research Institute, New Jersey Medical School, Rutgers, The State University of New Jersey, Newark, NJ, United States

K.J. Jensen
Research Center for Vitamins and Vaccines (CVIVA), Copenhagen S, Denmark

Jesper Kjærgaard
The Department of Paediatrics and Adolescent Medicine, Juliane Marie Centret, Rigshospitalet, Copenhagen University Hospital, Copenhagen, Denmark

Rosella Mechelli
Center for Experimental Neurological Therapies S. Andrea Hospital-site, Neurosciences, Mental Health, and Sensory Organs (NESMOS) Department, "Sapienza" University of Rome, Rome, Italy

Nicole L. Messina
Cancer & Disease Epigenetics and Infectious Diseases & Microbiology Research Groups, Murdoch Children's Research Institute; Department of Paediatrics, The University of Melbourne, Parkville, VIC, Australia

Emanuele Morena
Center for Experimental Neurological Therapies S. Andrea Hospital-site, Neurosciences, Mental Health, and Sensory Organs (NESMOS) Department, "Sapienza" University of Rome, Rome, Italy

Mihai G. Netea
Department of Internal Medicine and Radboud Center for Infectious Diseases, Radboud University Medical Center, Nijmegen, The Netherlands

Thomas Nørrelykke Nissen
Department of Paediatrics, Copenhagen University Hospital, Hvidovre, Denmark

Boris Novakovic
Cancer & Disease Epigenetics and Infectious Diseases & Microbiology Research Groups, Murdoch Children's Research Institute, Parkville, VIC, Australia

Roberta Reniè
Center for Experimental Neurological Therapies S. Andrea Hospital-site, Neurosciences, Mental Health, and Sensory Organs (NESMOS) Department, "Sapienza" University of Rome, Rome, Italy

A. Rieckmann
Research Center for Vitamins and Vaccines (CVIVA), Copenhagen S; OPEN, Institute of Clinical Research and Danish Institute of Advanced Science, University of Southern Denmark and Odense University Hospital, Odense, Denmark

Giovanni Ristori
Center for Experimental Neurological Therapies S. Andrea Hospital-site, Neurosciences, Mental Health, and Sensory Organs (NESMOS) Department, "Sapienza" University of Rome, Rome, Italy

Silvia Romano
Center for Experimental Neurological Therapies S. Andrea Hospital-site, Neurosciences, Mental Health, and Sensory Organs (NESMOS) Department, "Sapienza" University of Rome, Rome, Italy

Carmela Romano
Center for Experimental Neurological Therapies S. Andrea Hospital-site, Neurosciences, Mental Health, and Sensory Organs (NESMOS) Department, "Sapienza" University of Rome, Rome, Italy

Graham A.W. Rook
Centre for Clinical Microbiology, Department of Infection, UCL (University College London), London, United Kingdom

Marco Salvetti
Center for Experimental Neurological Therapies S. Andrea Hospital-site, Neurosciences, Mental Health, and Sensory Organs (NESMOS) Department, "Sapienza" University of Rome, Rome, Italy

Mona Singh
Special Centre for Molecular Medicine, Jawaharlal Nehru University, New Delhi, India

Nicola Vanacore
National Centre of Epidemiology, National Institute of Health, Rome, Italy

Vinod Yadav
Department of Microbiology, Central University of Haryana, Mahendergarh, India

INTRODUCTION

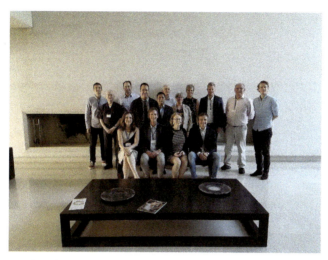

Attendees at the third biennial "BCG and TNF Signaling in the Treatment and Prevention of Autoimmune Diseases" conference held in Athens, Greece, October 7, 2017. Photo by Russell LaMontagne.

Left to right, first row: Marila Gennaro, Rutgers University; Nigel Curtis, University of Melbourne; Denise Faustman, Massachusetts General Hospital; Giovani Ristori, Sapienza University of Rome.

Left to right, second row: Bruce Bloom, Harvard School of Public Health; John Doupis, Iatriko Palaiou Faliro Medical Center; Gobardhan Das, University of Kwazulu-Nata; Hazel Dockrell, London School of Hygiene & Tropical Medicine.

Left to right, third row: Andreas Rieckmann, Statens Serum; Russell LaMontagne, Corinth Group; Graham Rook, University College London; Christine Stabell Benn, Statens Serum Institute; Thomas Nørrelykke Nissen, Copenhagen; Bob Glenister, Telpro; Rob Arts, Netherlands, Radboud Medical Center.

On October 7, 2017, the third biennial "BCG and TNF Signaling in the Treatment and Prevention of Autoimmune Diseases" conference was held in Athens, Greece. The first conference, held in London in 2013, served as the basis for the first edition of this book. Bacillus Calmette-Guérin (BCG) research has evolved enormously since that first conference and first edition. The first conference was a road map for BCG and autoimmunity, with ideas for moving forward and a glimpse into the potential of BCG. At the most recent conference in Athens, we heard updates on those early- and now late-stage clinical trials, gaining feedback and ideas from a diverse group of scientists from around the globe who are all interested in the ways BCG can play a role in the human immune system.

Barry Bloom from Harvard School of Public Health gave an overview of the public health status of BCG vaccination and current observations on immune response. Graham Rook from University College London revisited the "The Old Friends Hypothesis," the theory that autoimmune states are at least partly attributable to environmental change and the loss of mycobacterial infections, and discussed how BCG may promote immunoregulation. Rob Arts explained the work being done at the Radboud Medical Center in Holland to understand how cytokine production by BCG is correlated with induction of epigenetic changes.

Giovani Ristori from Sapienza University of Rome presented data from the ongoing BCG clinical trials in multiple sclerosis, which are aiming to prevent or delay disease onset in people with radiologically isolated syndrome (RIS). I updated the group on our Phase II BCG clinical trial program in type 1 diabetes, including new data showing a persistent response in type 1 diabetes and data on the impact of BCG on beneficial regulatory T-cell (Treg) populations.

Nigel Curtis from University of Melbourne presented an overview of the Melbourne Infant Study, a randomized controlled study of 1200 newborns to evaluate BCG for allergy and infection reduction up through 5 years of age. Thomas Nørrelykke Nissen of Copenhagen University Hospital gave an update on the 4000-patient Danish Calmette Study, in which infants were randomized 1:1 to neonatal BCG or no intervention and followed at 3 and 13 months to similarly look at the impact of BCG.

Finally, four talks examined the diverse and often gene-centered effects of BCG on the immune system, including important lessons we can learn from BCG and tuberculosis resistance and infections. Those speakers were Christine Stabell Benn and Andreas Rieckmann of Statens Serum Institute, Denmark; Hazel Dockrell of the London School of Hygiene & Tropical Medicine; Godardhan Das of the University of Kwazulu-Nata, India; and Marila Gennaro of Rutgers University.

We hope that this updated edition reflects the conference's energy and enthusiasm for the growing consensus that the BCG vaccine may be able to prevent and repair immune dysfunctions, and also, hopefully, offer a new perspective on the mechanisms involved.

Denise L. Faustman
Boston, MA, United States

CHAPTER 1

BCG: Its Impact on Tuberculosis and Relevance to Autoimmune Disease

Barry R. Bloom
Harvard T.H. Chan School of Public Health, Boston, MA, United States

Contents

ORIGINS

For centuries, TB was the largest cause of death in the world. Regrettably, TB currently remains the largest cause of death from any infectious disease, with about 10.5 million new cases and 1.5 million deaths each year.[1] The pathogens causing human TB are *Mycobacterium tuberculosis* (*Mtb*), transmitted by aerosol, and *Mycobacterium bovis,* transmitted by milk, which are even more virulent in humans. In 1908, Calmette and his associate, Guerin, working at the Institute Pasteur in Lille, sought to attenuate a virulent *M. bovis* strain by using the serial culture method devised by Pasteur, that we now know allows random mutations to accumulate. After 39 passages, they noticed a morphology change in some colonies, and after 230 passages, this strain (BCG), which had shown little toxicity and significant protection against TB in a variety of experimental animal models including nonhuman primates, was given for the first time in 1921 to a child at high risk for TB whose mother died of the disease and whose grandmother had active TB. That child survived to old age. Initially and for many years, BCG was given orally, but BCG is currently given intradermally. BCG remains the

The Value of BCG and TNF in Autoimmunity
https://doi.org/10.1016/B978-0-12-814603-3.00001-X

most widely utilized vaccine in the world, given to more than 100 million children a year and received by more than 4 billion to date worldwide. In animal models, CD4 and CD8 T cells appear to be necessary for protection, as are cytokines including IFN-γ and TNF-α, but the immunologic mechanisms underlying protection in humans remain unknown.

CURRENT BCG VACCINES

All BCG strains originated from the original Pasteur strain, but in the absence of modern methods for freezing, they were passaged under different conditions in many other laboratories (Fig. 1.1). BCG, like *Mtb* and *M. bovis,* grows slowly with a doubling time of about 24 h. Currently, the most widely used strains are Pasteur 1173P2, Danish SSI, Glaxo 1077, Tokyo 172-1, Russian BCG-I, Moreau RDJ, Montreal strain, and Tice strain, which is the only one licensed for use in the United States. With the exception of the Glaxo strain grown in liquid culture, the other strains are grown as pellicles on medium and harvested. The semidry mass is then broken up in a ball; milled into single bacilli, small clumps, and fragments; and are then lyophilized. One mg represents about 10^8 colony-forming units, and the portion of viable bacilli in most preparations ranges between 5% and 45%.[2–4]

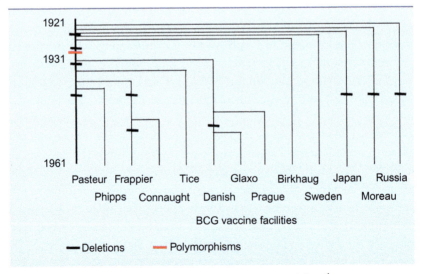

Fig. 1.1 Genealogy of BCG vaccine strains based on historical data.[4]

BCG AND PROTECTION AGAINST TB

Attenuating Mutations in BCG. The genomic DNA sequences of *Mtb*, *M. bovis*, and BCG are 99% homologous and colinear, indicating strong evolutionary similarities.[5] There are many polymorphisms and a number of large deletions, known as Regions of Difference (RD) that distinguish their sequences and virulence. The critical attenuating mutation is a deletion in RD1 that controls a set of secreted products of the Esx loci, which are essential for virulence and absent in all BCG strains. Two secreted proteins of the Esx-1 locus are major antigens of *Mtb* recognized by T cells and antibodies, and represent the basis of Elispot tests that can distinguish infection by *Mtb* from tuberculin skin test (TST)-positive conversions caused by BCG.[6] Three BCG strains (BCG Japan, BCG Glaxo, and BCG Moreau) have lost the ability to produce important lipid virulence factors, and those strains appear to have fewer adverse effects in clinical studies.[7] BCG vaccines are given intradermally generally close to the time of birth.

Protective Efficacy Against TB. Many randomized control trials, case-control trials, and observational studies have been carried out testing the protective efficacy of BCG vaccines against TB, and the results have varied enormously between trials in different countries. A recent systematic analysis of all randomized control trials has been carried out (Fig. 1.2).[8] The variation in protection ranged between 88% in the British Medical Research Council (MRC) trial to 0% in the Chingleput trial in South India. The most striking aspect of the variability is the geographic variance in protection; at higher latitudes, BCG had greater efficacy than in developing countries closer to the equator. In all Western European countries and the United States, the incidence of TB has been declining for a century, and it has been difficult to establish the impact of BCG in that context. For example, the Netherlands and the United States—which never employed BCG on a large scale but instead focused on screening for TST positivity and isoniazid preventive therapy, in contrast to the United Kingdom and Scandinavia, which instituted national BCG vaccine programs—had similar declines in incidence. BCG vaccine was more effective when given to young school children or infants. Although variation in many biological characteristics are found between different vaccine strains, for example in an ability to induce TST reactivity, the strain differences did not seem to be a major determinant of variation, and TST has not been a useful predictor of protective efficacy.

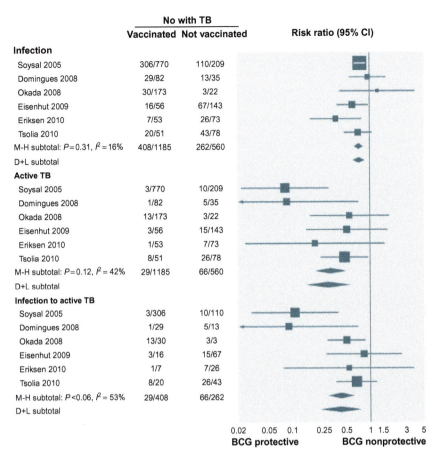

Fig. 1.2 Types of protection against *Mycobacterium tuberculosis* (TB) in children vaccinated with BCG. (*Modified from Roy A, Eisenhut M, Harris RJ, et al. Effect of BCG vaccination against Mycobacterium tuberculosis infection in children: systematic review and meta-analysis. BMJ. 2014;349(August 5):g4643. https://doi.org/10.1136/bmj.g4643.*)

Variability. Multiple hypothesis have been put forward to explain the wide variation between different trials, for example, the lack of critical protective antigens in *Mtb*, loss of potency by years of passage of strains, and different genetics of human populations. But the different effectiveness in latitudes is a clue to what is generally accepted to be the most likely explanation, namely interference by atypical or nontuberculous mycobacteria (NTM) in the environment. There are more than 300 species of NTM, and in animal studies, a gradient of protective efficacy is seen against *Mtb* challenge with *M. microti* and *M. kansasii* being as effective as

BCG, and others engendering little or no protection. In the South India trial, when testing for skin test reactivity to tuberculins derived from an *M. avian* strain, it was found that, by the age of 9, two-thirds of the children were positive, and 97% were positive by age 15. Hence prior exposure to cross-reactive antigens has an impact on the efficacy of BCG. It is unclear whether the failure to detect protection in individuals with prior exposure is due to protection already engendered by the environmental mycobacteria, such that the additional immunologic impact of BCG is reduced or negligible, or due to a blocking of the development of protective immunity by the NTM.

It is unclear how long protection induced by BCG persists. There is case-report evidence of children developing disseminated BCGosis a dozen years after immunization, so some organisms may persist in some individuals for long periods of time, but most evidence suggest that protective immunity wanes over the first decade or two after vaccination.

Safety. BCG has a remarkable record of safety over many decades of use in billions of children. After intradermal inoculation, erythema, induration, tenderness, and occasional ulceration may occur at the injection site, and a scar develops in most recipients. There may be swollen and tender axillary lymph nodes. The most serious and fortunately rare complication of BCG occurs in immunodeficient individuals, namely disseminated BCG disease that can be fatal. Thus, the use of BCG in HIV-infected infants not on antiretrovirals is contraindicated, and as a result of the success of antiretroviral treatment in preventing mother-to-child transmission of HIV, safety of BCG should become less of a problem.

Routes of immunization. In the initial human vaccination, BCG preparations in suspension were administered by the oral route on multiple days, the logic being that it would protect best by that route against oral ingestion of *M. bovis* in milk from infected cows. However, there were two problems: It required rather large amounts of bacilli to reproducibly generate skin test reactivity, and there was occasional cervical adenopathy. But Calmette was able to establish that there were detectable BCG bacilli in blood. In studies in rhesus macaques challenged by aerosol with *Mtb*, intravenous delivery was the most effective route at preventing lesions and bacillemia.[9,10] In humans, in the highly successful MRC trials, BCG was delivered percutaneously using multiple puncture devices and in some studies by aerosol, but there are no comparative data in humans to indicate which route of immunization is most effective in protecting against TB.

MECHANISM OF PROTECTION

The critical questions, the answers to which one would like to know in considering any vaccine, are: (i) What are the *necessary* and *sufficient* immunological conditions required to generate protective response? (ii) What are the antigens required to induce that response? And (iii) what is the best platform with which to generate that response? Regrettably, there is no perfect animal model faithful to the pattern of human TB or immune responses to it. Nevertheless, from animal studies it is clear that acquired immunity mediated by T cells is critical to protection against TB, and that both CD4 and CD8 T cells are essential. *Mtb* grows preferentially in macrophages, and macrophage activation by T cell-produced cytokines such as IFN-γ, TNFα, and IL-15 are critical. Although mouse macrophages are activated by cytokines to kill intracellular *Mtb* by production of nitric oxide, human monocyte-derived macrophages do not, killing *Mtb* by production of antimicrobial peptides including cathelicidin.[11]

Regulatory T cells (Tregs) are also involved as antiinflammatory and immunosuppressive cytokines such as IL-10. There is evidence in humans of a wide variety of cells in the innate immune system that may be involved at some level, including NK cells, γδT cells, HLA-E-restricted T cells, CD1-restricted T cells, and mucosal-associated invariant T cells (MAITS) found in lungs, but their role in protection remains unclear.[3]

One potentially important difference in the immune responses generated by *Mtb* and BCG in experimental animals may be noteworthy: *Mtb* is able to permeabilize the phagocytic vacuole and secrete antigens into the cytoplasm of antigen-presenting cells, thus generating cytotoxic T cells (CTL). BCG is unable to do so.[12]

After years of animal and human studies in which antibodies were found not to be involved in protection against TB, recent studies in vitro have suggested a possible role for antibodies in TB. A subset of individuals heavily exposed to *Mtb* but who were TST-negative and healthy, in fact, produce TB-specific IgG antibodies that can bind to the macrophage FcRγIII and activate macrophages to kill *Mtb* in vitro.[13]

Mtb encodes about 4000 proteins, and a very large number of antigens have been tested in animal in vitro models for stimulating immune responses and tested in protection. It is unlikely that any single protein or lipid antigen of *Mtb* will be found to be fully protective. It is more likely that multiple antigens, with epitopes recognized by different HLA types, will be required for protection. It is noteworthy that in the successful British MRC human trials of BCG against TB, an additional arm included *M. microti*, a mycobacterium that causes disease in the vole but not humans. Both *M. microti* and BCG produced comparable levels (~87%) of protection.

In summary, a wide range of immune responses are known to be involved in resistance and susceptibility to TB, and a number of responses are known to be necessary for protection. What is not known is which responses are sufficient to predict protection. And without biomarkers or correlates of protection, development and testing of new vaccine candidates will be severely limited.

NONSPECIFIC EFFECTS OF BCG

BCG has been found to have nonspecific immunological effects independent of its specific immune responses to *Mtb*. It is known to have adjuvant properties and to activate cells of the innate immune system to produce a wide variety of cytokines. In some trials, BCG immunization was found to be associated with major reductions in all-cause mortality or nonaccidental deaths of 20% to 60% in developing countries[14] and acute lower respiratory disease.[15] It has been reported that BCG reduced the appearance of brain lesions in early MS.[16] Local BCG instillation has now become the recommended treatment for superficial bladder cancers.[17] Understanding the mechanisms of the nonspecific immunologic effects of BCG may provide valuable insight into the mechanisms by which BCG influences autoimmune diseases.

SOME INTRIGUING CONNECTIONS WITH DIABETES

Although numerous small genetic differences exist between BCG vaccine strains that may lead to somewhat different responses to different antigens, the major deletions of pathogenesis genes in *M. bovis and M. tuberculosis* lead to an important immunological consequence. *Mtb* antigens are able to escape from phagocytic vesicles and enter the cytoplasm of macrophages, but BCG fails to do so. Because CD8 CTL are generated by peptides in the cytoplasm of infected antigen-presenting cells, *Mtb* generates both CTL and CD8 MHC Class I restricted CTL, necessary for protection against TB in experimental models. Thus, in the case of a CTL-mediated autoimmune disease, the question whether BCG vaccination is able to divert the autoimmune process mediated by autoreactive CTL either by stimulating Th2-helper cells for autoantibodies, inducing immunosuppressive cytokines such as IFN-β, IL-10, or TNFα, or amplifying Tregs that might reduce CTL activity remains an intriguing one that requires further study.

	Relative risk for active TB disease	Prevalence (%) (adults in 30 high TB burden countries)	Population attributable fraction (adults in 30 high TB burden countries)
HIV	21	0.9	15
Undernutrition	3.2	12	21
Diabetes	3.1	8.5	15
Alcohol misuse	2.9	4.0	7.0
Smoking	1.9	19	15
Indoor air pollution	1.4	53	17

Fig. 1.3 Population attributable fractions for risk factors for tuberculosis.[1]

Among major risk factors for acquiring clinical TB beyond undernutrition, diabetes is second only to HIV as a major risk factor, encompassing the major population of potential susceptibles worldwide in the future (Fig. 1.3),[1] the underlying mechanisms of this association remain unclear. An interesting possible association of an immune response to mycobacterial antigens, which may merely represent coincidence, exists in studies of lepromatous leprosy. In the disseminated form of the disease, in which T cells failed to respond to antigens of *M. leprae*, there was evidence for the presence of T regulatory cells that were restricted by HLA-DQ.[18] The major genetic associations for acquiring type 1 diabetes involves MHC Class II haplotypes, the most at-risk being the DRB1-DQA1-DQB1 haplotype. A reduction in the functional capacity of Tregs has been reported in T1D.[19] In the simplest case, in healthy individuals, autoimmune T cells are either clonally deleted or controlled by Treg cells, or reduced by proinflammatory cytokines such as IFN-β and IL-10 that suppress CTL responses. If there are haplotypes in which Tregs are effectively unable to control pancreatic β-cell-specific CD8 CTL, autoimmune damage to the pancreas would result. The original studies deleting the gene for PD-1, the marker for programmed cell death, revealed that anti–PD-1 antibodies in normal mice led to a variety of autoimmune diseases.[20] The hypothesis that autoimmune responses are normally regulated in healthy humans is supported by recent observations on the outcomes of the checkpoint inhibitor, anti–PD-1, in the treatment of human cancers. In a number of these patients, de novo autoimmune diabetes occurred in adults above age 55, in which both antipancreas antibodies and CD8-reactive T cells were present,[21] consistent with the interpretation that the autoreactive cells were present but under regulatory control until suppressed by the anti-PD-1 antibodies. That regulatory control may, in part, be mediated by IL-10.[22] Although this may lead to renewed anticancer CTL activity, it may also precipitate activation of autoimmune responses.

REFERENCES

1. WHO. *Global TB report.* Geneva: WHO; 2016.
2. Bloom BR, Fine PEM. The BCG experience: implications for future vaccines against tuberculosis. In: Bloom BR, ed. *Tuberculosis: Pathogenesis, Protection, and Control.* Washington, DC: ASM Press; 1994:531–557.
3. Hanekom W. Tuberculosis vaccines. In: Bloom BR, Lambert P-H, eds. *The Vaccine Book.* New York, NY: Elsevier Publishing; 2017:363–383.
4. Behr M. BCG-different strains, different vaccines? *Lancet Infect Dis.* 2002;2(2):86–92.
5. Tran V, Liu J, Behr MA. BCG vaccines. *Microbiol Spectr.* 2014;2(1):MGM2-0028-2013.
6. Pai M, Zwerling A, Menzies D. Systematic review: T-cell-based assays for the diagnosis of latent tuberculosis infection: an update. *Ann Intern Med.* 2008;149(3):177–184.
7. Lotte A, Wasz-Hockert O, Poisson N, Dumitrescu N, Verron M, Couvet E. BCG complications. Estimates of the risks among vaccinated subjects and statistical analysis of their main characteristics. *Adv Tuberc Res.* 1984;21:107–193.
8. Roy A, Eisenhut M, Harris RJ, et al. Effect of BCG vaccination against Mycobacterium tuberculosis infection in children: systematic review and meta-analysis. *BMJ.* 2014;349(August 5):g4643. https://doi.org/10.1136/bmj.g4643.
9. Barclay RW, Anacker RL, Brehmer M, Leif W, Ribi E. Aerosol-induced tuberculosis in subhuman primates and the course of the disease after intravenous BCG vaccination. *Infect Immun.* 1970;2:574–582.
10. Anacker RL, Brehmer W, Barclay WR, et al. Superiority of intravenously administered BeG and BCG cell walls in protecting rhesus monkeys (*Macaca mulatta*) against airborne tuberculosis. *Z Immunitatsforsch Exp Klin Immunol.* 1972;143(4):363–376.
11. Liu PT, Stenger S, Li H, et al. Toll-like receptor triggering of a vitamin D-mediated human antimicrobial response. *Science.* 2006;311(5768):1770–1773.
12. Flynn JL, Goldstein MM, Triebold KJ, Koller B, Bloom BR. Major histocompatibility complex class I-restricted T cells are required for resistance to *Mycobacterium tuberculosis* infection. *Proc Natl Acad Sci USA.* 1992;89(24):12013–12017.
13. Lu LL, Chung AW, Rosebrock T, et al. Functional role for antibodies in tuberculosis. *Cell.* 2016;167(2):433–443.
14. Higgins JP, Soares-Weiser K, López-López JA, et al. Association of BCG, DTP, and measles containing vaccines with childhood mortality: systematic review. *BMJ.* 2016;355:i5170.
15. Hollm-Delgado MG, Stuart EA, Black RE. Acute lower respiratory infection among Bacille Calmette-Guerin (BCG)-vaccinated children. *Pediatrics.* 2013;133(1):e73–81.
16. Ristori G, Romano S, Cannoni S, et al. Effects of Bacille Calmette-Guerin after the first demyelinating event in the CNS. *Neurology.* 2014;82(1):41–48.
17. Sylvester RJ, van der Meijdan AP, Lamm DL. Intravesical bacillus Calmette-Guerin reduces the risk of progression in patients with superficial bladder cancer: a meta-analysis of the published results of randomized clinical trials. *J Urol.* 2002;168(5):1964–1970.
18. Noble JA, Valdes AM. Genetics of the HLA region in the prediction of type 1 diabetes. *Curr Diab Rep.* 2011;11(6):533–542.
19. Hull C, Peakman M, Tree T. Regulatory T cell dysfunction in type 1 diabetes: what's broken and how can we fix it? *Diabetologia.* 2017;60:1839–1850. https://doi.org/10.1007/s00125-017-4377-1. [Epub ahead of print.].

20. Nishimura H, Nose M, Hiai H, Minato N, Honjo T. Development of lupus-like autoimmune diseases by disruption of the PD-1 gene encoding an ITIM motif-carrying immunoreceptor. *Immunity*. 1999;11(2):141–151.
21. Hughes J, Vutattu N, Sznol M, et al. Precipitation of autoimmune diabetes with anti-PD-1 immunotherapy. *Diabetes Care*. 2015;38(4):e55–7.
22. Said EA, Dupuy FP, Trautmann L, et al. Programmed death-1-induced interleukin-10 production by monocytes impairs CD4+ T cell activation during HIV infection. *Nat Med*. 2010;16(4):452–459.

CHAPTER 2

The Potential of TNF Induction From BCG for the Treatment of Type 1 Diabetes

Denise L. Faustman
Director of Immunobiology, Massachusetts General Hospital, Boston, MA, United States
Associate Professor of Medicine, Harvard Medical School, Boston, MA, United States

Contents

In type 1 diabetes, insulin–autoreactive T cells mediate destruction of the pancreatic beta cells that produce insulin, leading to insulin deficiency, hyperglycemia, and the need for lifelong insulin injections. Despite insulin treatment, many patients with type 1 diabetes will develop disease-related microvascular and macrovascular complications, underscoring the need for new, effective interventions that address the underlying causes of the disease.

The predominant cause of type 1 diabetes is autoreactive T cells directed to diverse insulin-secreting islet cell proteins. In addition, type 1 diabetes and other forms of autoimmunity appear to be driven by an immune imbalance due to too few or poorly functioning Tregs, which are a subtype of T lymphocytes that help maintain tolerance to selfantigens and suppress or quiet the immune response, as well as too many effector T cells (Teffs) or cytotoxic T cells.[1] Specifically, at the tissue site in these autoimmune diseases, there are too few Tregs and too many Teffs or cytotoxic T cells.

The Value of BCG and TNF in Autoimmunity
https://doi.org/10.1016/B978-0-12-814603-3.00002-1

Preclinical and clinical evidence suggests that induction of TNF using the BCG vaccine or agonism of TNFR2 using novel antibodies may provide a pathway to targeted and selective destruction of the autoreactive T cells in type 1 diabetes.[2–4] Further, this treatment approach may also alter the abnormal tissue microenvironment in autoimmunity and convert it to a nondisease state by inducing Tregs that suppress pathologic T cells.

TNF can directly and selectively kill the autoreactive T cells both in diabetes prone nonobese diabetic (NOD) mice as well as in humans with type 1 diabetes.[5–7] Clinical trials in type 1 diabetes are currently investigating this strategy, especially as it relates to medications—notably the BCG vaccine—that induce elevation of TNF levels to both kill autoreactive autoreactive T cells and expand Tregs. Long-term follow up the BCG treated patients from the Phase I clinical trial showed a lasting and statistically significant change in blood sugar as measured by HbA1c beginning a year three and maintained beyond five additional years of follow up.

This chapter discusses in more detail the role of the TNF pathway and the use of TNF inducers such as BCG or TNFR2 agonists as treatments for established type 1 diabetes, focusing on recent human data and supporting data from other autoimmune diseases.

SIGNALING DEFECTS IN THE TNF PATHWAY MAKE AUTOREACTIVE T CELLS VULNERABLE TO APOPTOSIS AFTER TNF ELEVATIONS FROM BCG

The rationale behind targeting the TNF pathway in type 1 diabetes is based on work that first identified signaling defects in the NFκB pathway of autoimmune mice[8,9] and then showed in mice and humans that these intracellular signaling errors in autoreactive T cells make the cells selectively vulnerable to death upon exposure to or induction of TNF.[5,7,10,11] Data similarly shows that TNFR2 agonism can effectively and selectively kill insulin-autoreactive CD8 T cells in blood samples taken from patients with type 1 diabetes.[5] Indeed, the mycobacteria tubulosis bacilli itself also modifies the host macrophage's trimeric membrane TNF, the nature ligand for TNFR2 Tregs for expansion.

What exactly is this signaling error, and why does it make autoreactive T cells—but not normal T cells—vulnerable to TNF-induced apoptosis? In normal T cells, TNF activates the proteasomal cleavage of NFκB from IKBα. After cleavage, NFκB enters the nucleus and initiates transcription of an array of antiapoptotic proteins that counteract the proapoptotic effects of TNF.[12] Thus, NFκB activation in normal cells is protective, preventing cells from death upon TNF exposure.

Conversely, in type 1 diabetes and some other forms of autoimmunity, this process is disrupted. Genetic or functional defects prevent transcription factor signaling in the NFκB pathway, thereby preventing this prolife survival factor from entering the nucleus to express prosurvival genes. NFκB cannot be activated to counteract TNF-induced apoptosis, leaving the cell vulnerable to death. In experiments performed in vitro, incubating TNF with blood samples from patients with type 1 diabetes and other autoimmune diseases known to have defects in the NFκB pathway led to death of a subpopulation of autoreactive CD8 T cells but not CD4 T cells.[5]

Soluble TNF can bind to both TNF receptor 1 (TNFR1) and TNFR2. Preferential binding is toward TNFR1, which is ubiquitously expressed, whereas TNFR2 has more limited cellular expression in the normal immune system and is primarily expressed on T cells, subsets of neurons, and a few other cell types such as Tregs and diseased cytotoxic T cells. TNFR1's more ubiquitous expression, which correlates with toxicity data, even in baboons, suggests that TNFR2 agonism would be expected to have a better toxicology profile.

The natural ligand for TNFR2 is trimeric membrane TNF, most often expressed on monocytes. The engagement of TNF with its receptors results in contrasting responses, depending on the receptor. In nondiseased cells, TNFR1 is linked to cell death pathways. Therefore, sole engagement of TNFR1 results in cell death. In contrast, sole engagement of TNFR2 causes normal CD8 T cells to proliferate because TNFR2 intracellularly lacks a death receptor. This paradoxical response between engagement with TNFR1 and TNFR2 is due to both the activation state of the T cells and that the TNF receptors have very different TNF-signaling pathways (i.e., the TNFR1 intracellular domain is a cell death domain, whereas the TNFR2 intracellular domain is linked to NFκB expansion).

In diseased CD8 T cells from autoimmune patients (all who express TNFR2), TNF or TNFR2 agonism causes selective cell death through an altered signaling pathway. This ability of TNF or TNFR2 engagement to be selective for CD8-driven cell death was functionally tested in the human disease setting of type 1 diabetes and other autoimmune diseases. Fresh autoimmune CD8 T cells from autoimmune patients were incubated with either TNF, TNFR1-agonistic antibodies, or TNFR2-agonistic antibodies. The human autoimmune data were clear: only TNFR2 agonists, but not

TNFR1 agonists, had the ability to target and kill the autoreactive T cells from diverse human autoimmune diseases, including cytotoxic T cells in type 1 diabetes, as well as autoimmune cells in multiple sclerosis, Graves' disease, Crohn's disease, and other forms of autoimmunity.[5] In patients with type 1 diabetes, the subpopulation of T cells vulnerable to TNF or TNFR2 agonist-induced death was traceable to insulin-autoreactive CD8 T cells.[5]

Additionally, murine autoimmune data show that TNF, TNF induction, and TNFR2 agonism all relieve the burden of autoreactive cells by selectively inducing cell death and also preventing disease transfer.[12,13]

Overall, these data suggest that signaling defects through the TNF pathway, whether through NFκB or activators of NFκB, such as the proteasome complex and the ubiquitination process, may provide an important opportunity for intervention in type 1 diabetes.

TNF INDUCTION AND TNFR2 AGONISM TRIGGER TREG EXPANSION

In addition to eliminating autoreactive cells, TNF induction or TNFR2 agonism may work through a second mechanism by triggering the induction or expansion of Tregs. Tregs are a subset of CD4 T cells that help to prevent or treat autoimmunity by maintaining self-tolerance, immune homeostasis, and suppression of cytotoxic T cells.[1] However, clinical application of Tregs in autoimmunity has previously been hampered by the difficulty in obtaining and safely administering sufficient quantities of Tregs, whether generated in vitro or stimulated in vivo, to be effective. Recent studies, however, suggest that there may now be a way forward, at least in certain forms of autoimmunity.

In humans with long-standing type 1 diabetes, repeat BCG administration (two doses) induced proliferation of Tregs in a phase I clinical trial,[14] which appeared to contribute to early clinical benefits, including suppression of disease and transient restoration of low-level insulin secretion.

Similar to BCG vaccinations, TNFR2 agonism induces proliferation of Tregs in the mouse[15] and in vitro in humans.[4] TNFR2-expressing Tregs are highly suppressive and appear to be the most suppressive Tregs identified to date in the mouse and human.[16–19] TNFR2 agnonism using antibodies or transmembrane TNF induces IL2R (CD25), TNF, and TRAF2 expression, all of which are elements of the TNFR2-signaling pathway for Treg expansion.[4] Interestingly, the Tregs observed after expansion through TNFR2 agonism in a study by Okubo et al. are a homogenous population, contrasting with the heterogeneous population observed when a TNFR1 agonist is used to trigger expansion in human cell cultures.[4] This homogeneity is important, because heterogeneous progeny are capable of releasing proinflammatory cytokines and can also include cell populations with antagonistic properties. Further, the Tregs in the same study exerted an immunosuppressive function that may be beneficial in type 1 diabetes.

On an historical note, it is important to point out that the triggering of TNF release by the host immune system after BCG vaccination or tuberculosis exposure defines the innate immune response. The ability of BCG or other select microbial pathogens to trigger systemic "cachectin" (which was renamed TNF after cloning) release is well documented.[20] Although many immune cells can produce and release TNF after BCG exposure, macrophages, in general, release the largest amount of this cytokine when exposed.

TREATING TYPE 1 DIABETES IN THE NOD MOUSE WITH BCG OR TNFR2 AGONISM

Historical evidence supports the premise that autoimmune-prone NOD mice with both type 1 diabetes and Sjögren's syndrome are amenable to treatments with adjuvants that stimulate TNF, such as BCG or its heat-inactivated equivalent, complete Freund's adjuvant (CFA). Like many other interventions, BCG and CFA can prevent type 1 diabetes onset if administered to young NOD mice.[21–25] What distinguishes BCG and CFA from many other forms of immunotherapy in mice, however, is that these agents cannot only stop new-onset diabetes but also reverse end-stage diabetes.[11,26]

In animal models, double dosing of BCG was more effective than single dosing in preventing diabetes onset in NOD mice.[27] In addition, for BCG or CFA to be effective in the NOD mouse model, the immune adjuvant needed to be administered after the autoimmune disease had started the attack in the pancreas. If BCG, CFA, or TNF was administered at birth in NOD mice, disease prevention did not occur, and some data have shown that BCG administered at birth in the mouse can accelerate disease expression.[28] NOD mouse data also show that, in mice administered CFA, BCG, or TNF, upregulated Tregs appeared—a potential benefit due to the possible disease-reversing effects of these immune quieting cells.[29,30]

Unlike many other "cures" of type 1 diabetes in mice, BCG or CFA prevented or reversed type 1 diabetes while imposing little or no toxicity. Although the mechanism for efficacy is mediated through TNF, systemic toxicity prevents the use of direct TNF administration at high doses in the human. However, TNF induction with a safe vaccine such as the BCG vaccine or via TNFR2 agonism may be a way to correct signaling defects and safely address autoimmunity through selective destruction of autoreactive T cells and induction of Tregs that suppress cytotoxic T cells.

THE BCG VACCINE IN TYPE 1 DIABETES: STRAIN DIFFERENCES, DOSE, AND TIMING FOR MAXIMAL EFFICACY?

In the past decade, interest in the nearly century-old tuberculosis vaccine, BCG, has been revived for potential therapeutic uses in new indications, including type 1 diabetes and other types of autoimmunity.

BCG has an excellent long-standing record of safety and tolerability. The most common adverse event, which is still rare, is suppurative lymphadenitis, a reaction that is self-limiting and not treated but is an irritating consequence of a local lymph node response. The BCG vaccine's main appeal for investigations in the treatment of autoimmunity is its ability to induce TNF. BCG contains the avirulent tuberculosis strain *Mycobacterium bovis* and was first introduced into humans in 1921 as a vaccine to prevent tuberculosis. Since its introduction, an estimated 3 billion people worldwide have received the vaccine. However, because of the declining incidence of tuberculosis in Europe and the United States, routine BCG vaccination has been discontinued at these sites. In contrast, the BCG vaccine is broadly and uniformly administered in developing countries.

In type 1 diabetes, the potential benefit of BCG vaccinations was first demonstrated in the NOD rodent model, as previously discussed. TNF induction with CFA or BCG in the NOD mouse reversed advanced disease by killing disease-causing autoimmune cells and restoring insulin secretion.[11,26] CFA and BCG are similar products in that they contain *Mycobacteria*; CFA contains inactivated *Mycobacterium,* whereas BCG contains avirulent *Mycobacterium* that has historically undergone many rounds of in vitro selection to decrease virulence in humans. CFA is a research tool, whereas BCG is a clinical product suitable for use in the human.

Recent human clinical trials in type 1 diabetes and multiple sclerosis in adults who were administered the BCG vaccine show therapeutic promise, even after disease onset or in long-established autoimmunity,[14,31–34] although early trials, conducted without an awareness of strains nor necessary dosing, showed variable effects.

In an early, uncontrolled trial by Shehadeh et al., which included 17 patients who were newly diagnosed with type 1 diabetes, a single dose of BCG led to a temporary remission in 11 patients (65%).[35] This study used the Moreau strain of BCG. However, subsequent controlled clinical trials using a single low dose of BCG as the TICE strain and epidemiologic studies in children with new onset type 1 diabetes[36–38] did not show a benefit to BCG vaccination when followed for 6 month, 1 year, or 2 years, time points that, in multiple sclerosis, are too short to show the therapeutic reversal or halt of autoimmunity in humans.

The reason for the negative findings may be due to insufficient (i.e., single) dosing, as well as the use of different BCG strains such as TICE, which has low efficacy even in mouse studies. Interestingly, in the early human study by Shehadeh et al. in which single dosing of BCG led to temporary remission of new-onset type 1 diabetes in 11 of 17 patients, an older BCG strain was used that is known to induce strong host TNF responses.[35] In contrast, the later type 1 diabetes studies frequently used the TICE strain of BCG, which has lower efficacy in terms of NFκB induction and TNF production, as well as lower protective responses against tuberculosis.[39,40] BCG's mechanism of action was not known until approximately 10 years ago, and it was not appreciated that strain differences might impact efficacy, nor that longer follow-up of subjects might be essential. Moreover, with a more advanced understanding of the mechanism of action of BCG, it is now possible to pair biomarkers for early indications of efficacy in clinical trials, use the correct strain of BCG, and be aware of the time period subjects must be followed for these permanet effects of the vaccine.

About a decade after BCG was first studied in humans with type 1 diabetes, a double-blind, placebo-controlled phase I trial of repeat BCG vaccination was conducted in adults with long-standing type 1 diabetes (mean duration of diabetes: 15.3 years) at a single center in the United States.[14] Six type 1 diabetic subjects were randomly assigned to BCG or placebo (two injections spaced 4 weeks apart) and were compared with self, a healthy paired control ($n = 6$), or reference subjects with ($n = 57$) or without ($n = 16$) type 1 diabetes (depending on the outcome measure) over a 20-week period. Within several weeks, repeat BCG vaccinations led to a large increase in dead insulin-autoreactive T cells entering into the circulation (i.e., selectively eliminated insulin-autoreactive T cells) and transiently induced beneficial Tregs for 4 to 6 weeks after BCG administration. In these human studies, the Connaught strain of BCG (manufactured by Sanofi) was utilized. These findings were not only seen in the BCG-treated patients but also in one placebo-treated patient who developed an acute infection with the Epstein-Barr virus (EBV) after enrollment. EBV infection is known to trigger robust release of TNF. Therefore, the response of the participant who unexpectedly developed EBV underscores the benefits of triggering innate immunity[20] in long-standing type 1 diabetes.[41] In two BCG-treated subjects and the one EBV-infected subject, treatment transiently restored a small amount of insulin production as measured by C-peptide levels and as detected by an ultrasensitive assay. As expected from the long safety history of the BCG vaccine, no major adverse events were reported.

This trial was the first to demonstrate that, by transiently arresting the autoimmune response that underlies type 1 diabetes, BCG treatment or EBV infection can pave the way for some degree of transcient, albeit non-clinically significant, C-peptide restoration even in patients with a long duration of type 1 diabetes (>10 years duration). Long-term follow-up of phase I participants continues, including analysis of patients in the placebo arm who have now received BCG in an open-label crossover portion of the study. A randomized, placebo-controlled phase II trial is also currently underway, with an endpoint of a >10% lowering of HbA1c values. Data from multiple sclerosis trials with BCG show that clinically significant immune alterations after BCG administration may take time to occur.[31] Therefore, a trial duration of 5 years has been selected for the phase II type 1 diabetes study as a clinical outcome, not just a biomarker outcome, is desired.

It is interesting to note that the positive findings from the phase I type 1 diabetes trial are consistent with trials of BCG vaccination in multiple sclerosis, an autoimmune disease in which autoreactive T cells are also susceptible to TNF-triggered cell death. In trials conducted in Italy, BCG vaccination was found to decrease multiple sclerosis disease activity and prevent progression of brain lesions in patients with relapsing-remitting disease.[32,33] These studies were followed by a double-blind, placebo-controlled phase II trial testing BCG vaccination in subjects with early symptoms of multiple sclerosis (i.e., clinically isolated syndromes [CIS]), but who had not yet been definitively diagnosed with advanced multiple sclerosis.[31,34] A single dose of BCG was administered to 33 subjects, whereas an additional 40 subjects received the placebo. Vaccinated subjects were significantly less likely to develop lesions within 6 months of vaccination, and the number of T1-hypointense lesions was lower in the BCG group at 6, 12, and 18 months. Further, at the end of 5 years, 58% of subjects who received BCG did not progress to multiple sclerosis, compared with 30% of those who received the placebo. Overall, clinical benefits after BCG administration in new-onset multiple sclerosis were durable and were even enhanced at 5 years.[31] There were no major adverse events, and the frequency of all adverse events did not differ between treated and placebo groups. The benefits of BCG vaccination in multiple sclerosis continue to be investigated in a phase III clinical trial.

Long-term follow-up of the Phase I, BCG-treated, type 1 diabetic subjects showed results consistent with the MS trial results. Beginning after the third year of treatment, all patients in the BCG-treated group showed lasting, statistically significant, and clinically relevant improvements in HbA1c to near-normal levels (BCG 6.18+/-.34 vs placebo 7.07+/-.41, p = 0.002), extending beyond the next five years of monitoring[53]. In addition to improvements in blood sugar, the BCG-treated patients showed no adverse advents such as hypoglycemia.

DOES BCG WORK THROUGH OTHER PATHWAYS THAN TRANSMEMBRANE TNF AND TNFR2 RECEPTOR?

TNFR2 Agonism as a Treatment for Type 1 Diabetes

Unlike TNF induction through the BCG vaccine, which is currently advancing in human trials, TNFR2 agonism as a treatment for type 1 diabetes is still under preclinical investigation, with studies showing benefits in various autoimmune settings. As previously mentioned, from the tuberculosis field it is known that many of the immune-modulatory effects of myocbacteria are through induced host transmemberane TNF in monocytes and the induction of potent surrounding Tregs through this natural ligand for the most potent Tregs, TNFR2+ Tregs.[42]

As mentioned earlier, a TNFR2 agonist has been shown to selectively kill autoreactive T cells from patients with type 1 diabetes in culture.[5] Further in vitro studies show that a Treg activation defect in type 1 diabetes can be corrected with TNFR2 agonism.[43] Activated Tregs (aTregs) prevent or halt various forms of autoimmunity. Okubo et al. have shown that patients with type 1 diabetes have elevated numbers of resting Tregs (rTregs, CD4(+)CD25(+)Foxp3(+)CD45RA) and a decrease in aTregs (CD4(+)CD25(+)Foxp3(+)CD45RO) compared with controls ($n = 55$ type 1 diabetics, $n = 45$ controls, $P = .01$), which is associated with a trend for less residual C-peptide secretion from the pancreas ($P = .08$) and poorer HbA1c control ($P = .03$). TNFR2 agonism was used as a method for stimulating conversion of rTregs to aTregs, which corrected the activation defect.

Further, TNFR2 agonism was superior to standard protocols and to TNF in proliferating Tregs. TNFR2 agonist-expanded Tregs were homogeneous and functionally potent by virtue of suppressing autologous cytotoxic T cells in a dose-dependent manner comparable to controls. Thus, targeting the TNFR2 receptor for Treg expansion, at least in vitro, demonstrates a means to correct the activation defect in type 1 diabetes.[44]

Often when the benefit of TNF induction through BCG is described, it is hard to reconcile with the vast autoimmune literature that shows some subsets of autoimmune subjects benefit from anti-TNF therapy, such as those with rheumatoid arthritis. Previously, it was presumed that anti-TNF therapies "took away" TNF as their mechanism for clinical benefit. New data perhaps explain this paradox. From the rheumatoid arthritis literature, it is known that the anti-TNF therapies infliximab and adalimumab induce Tregs in autoimmune patients. These drugs are antibodies that bind TNF. Another approved drug for rheumatoid arthritis is etanercept, a soluble TNFR2 antibody receptor-linked antibody. Etanercept does not induce Tregs in vivo.[45] In culture, human Tregs expanded with TNF are potent Tregs.[18,44–49] It is now appreciated that the therapeutic anti-TNF antibody adalimumab induces Tregs in vivo, but by binding preferentially to membrane surface TNF with trimerization that induces TNFR2 on Treg cells, both in vivo and in vitro.[50] Because TNFR2 Tregs are the most suppressive Tregs known to exist naturally, and are also the abundant Treg subtype in cancer-conferring suppression, this means anti-TNF therapy is not working through TNF reduction but rather through TNF trimerization and TNFR2 induction of potent Tregs. Thus, adalimumab is expanding functional and potent TNFR2 Tregs well with potent suppressive activity.[50]

Recent data show that TNFR2 agonism restricts the pathogenicity of CD8 T cells in murine colitis.[51] Additionally, a TNFR2 agonist expands potent host Treg cells in vitro, and also protects in vivo from acute graft versus host disease in a mouse.[44] In the human, exogenous TNFR2 activation protects from acute graft-versus-host disease (GVHD) via host Treg cell expansion.[52]

CONCLUSIONS

Administration of agents that induce TNF (i.e., BCG) or agonize TNFR2 is a new treatment strategy being investigated for the treatment of type 1 diabetes. TNF induction and TNFR2 agonism have been associated with the selective death of autoreactive T cells, induction of Tregs, and even early clinical signs, in vivo, of pancreatic islet function restoration. The use of BCG as an immune intervention in current type 1 diabetes treatment trials is based on its potential to eliminate autoreactive T cells, induce a protective host TNF response (including induction of Tregs), and possibly provide long-term modulation of the immuno-inflammatory profile in patients who are vaccinated. Long-term follow up of type 1 diabetes patients treated with BCG showed durable, statistically significant changes in blood sugar beginning at year three of treatment.

REFERENCES

1. Miyara M, Gorochov G, Ehrenstein M, Musset L, Sakaguchi S, Amoura Z. Human FoxP3+ regulatory T cells in systemic autoimmune diseases. *Autoimmun Rev.* 2011;10:744–755.
2. Faustman DL. TNF BCG, and the proteasome in autoimmunity: an overview of the pathways & results of a phase I study in type 1 diabetes. In: Faustman DL, ed. *The Value of BCG and TNF in Autoimmunity.* Boston, MA: Academic Press; 2014:81–104.
3. Faustman D, Davis M. TNF receptor 2 pathway: drug target for autoimmune diseases. *Nat Rev Drug Discov.* 2010;9:482–493.
4. Okubo Y, Mera T, Wang L, Faustman DL. Homogeneous expansion of human T regulatory cells via tumor necrosis factor receptor 2. *Sci Rep.* 2013;3:3153.
5. Ban L, Zhang J, Wang L, Kuhtreiber W, Burger D, Faustman DL. Selective death of autoreactive T cells in human diabetes by TNF or TNF receptor 2 agonism. *Proc Natl Acad Sci USA.* 2008;105:13644–13649.
6. Christen U, Wolfe T, Mohrle U, et al. A dual role for TNF-alpha in type 1 diabetes: islet-specific expression abrogates the ongoing autoimmune process when induced late but not early during pathogenesis. *J Immunol.* 2001;166:7023–7032.
7. Qin HY, Chaturvedi P, Singh B. In vivo apoptosis of diabetogenic T cells in NOD mice by IFN-gamma/TNF-alpha. *Int Immunol.* 2004;16:1723–1732.
8. Hayashi T, Faustman D. NOD mice are defective in proteasome production and activation of NF-kappaB. *Mol Cell Biol.* 1999;19:8646–8659.
9. Hayashi T, Faustman D. Essential role of HLA-encoded proteasome subunits in NF-kB activation and prevention of TNF-a induced apoptosis. *J Biol Chem.* 2000;275:5238–5247.
10. Christen U, Von Herrath MG. Apoptosis of autoreactive CD8 lymphocytes as a potential mechanism for the abrogation of type 1 diabetes by islet-specific TNF-alpha expression at a time when the autoimmune process is already ongoing. *Ann N Y Acad Sci.* 2002;958:166–169.
11. Ryu S, Kodama S, Ryu K, Schoenfeld DA, Faustman DL. Reversal of established autoimmune diabetes by restoration of endogenous beta cell function. *J Clin Invest.* 2001;108:63–72.
12. Kodama S, Davis M, Faustman DL. The therapeutic potential of tumor necrosis factor for autoimmune disease: a mechanistically based hypothesis. *Cell Mol Life Sci.* 2005;62:1850–1862.
13. Kuhtreiber WM, Hayashi T, Dale EA, Faustman DL. Central role of defective apoptosis in autoimmunity. *J Mol Endocrinol.* 2003;31:373–399.
14. Faustman DL, Wang L, Okubo Y, et al. Proof-of-concept, randomized, controlled clinical trial of bacillus-Calmette-Guerin for treatment of long-term type 1 diabetes. *PLoS One.* 2012;7:e41756.

15. Chen X, Baumel M, Mannel DN, Howard OM, Oppenheim JJ. Interaction of TNF with TNF receptor type 2 promotes expansion and function of mouse CD4+CD25+ T regulatory cells. *J Immunol.* 2007;179:154–161.

16. Chen X, Subleski JJ, Hamano R, Howard OMZ, Wiltrout RH, Oppenheim JJ. Co-expression of TNFR2 and CD25 identifies more of the functional CD4(+)FOXP3(+) regulatory T cells in human peripheral blood. *Eur J Immunol.* 2010;40:1099–1106.

17. Chen X, Subleski JJ, Kopf H, Howard OM, Mannel DN, Oppenheim JJ. Cutting edge: expression of TNFR2 defines a maximally suppressive subset of mouse CD4+CD25+-FoxP3+ T regulatory cells: applicability to tumor-infiltrating T regulatory cells. *J Immunol.* 2008;180:6467–6471.

18. Chen X, Wu X, Zhou Q, Howard OM, Netea MG, Oppenheim JJ. TNFR2 is critical for the stabilization of the CD4+Foxp3+ regulatory T cell phenotype in the inflammatory environment. *J Immunol.* 2013;190:1076–1084.

19. Govindaraj C, Scalzo-Inguanti K, Madondo M, et al. Impaired Th1 immunity in ovarian cancer patients is mediated by TNFR2+ Tregs within the tumor microenvironment. *Clin Immunol.* 2013;149:97–110.

20. Rahman MM, McFadden G. Modulation of tumor necrosis factor by microbial pathogens. *PLoS Pathog.* 2006;2:e4.

21. Harada M, Kishimoto Y, Makino S. Prevention of overt diabetes and insulitis in NOD mice by a single BCG vaccination. *Diabetes Res Clin Pract.* 1990;8:85–89.

22. Sadelain MWJ, Hui-Yu Q, Lauzon J, Singh B. Prevention of type I diabetes in NOD mice by adjuvant immunotherapy. *Diabetes.* 1990;39:583–589.

23. Sadelain MW, Qin HY, Sumoski W, Parfrey N, Singh B, Rabinovitch A. Prevention of diabetes in the BB rat by early immunotherapy using Freund's adjuvant. *J Autoimmun.* 1990;3:671–680.

24. McInerney MF, Pek SB, Thomas DW. Prevention of insulitis and diabetes onset by treatment with complete Freund's adjuvant in NOD mice. *Diabetes.* 1991;40:715–725.

25. Qin HY, Sadelain MW, Hitchon C, Lauzon J, Singh B. Complete Freund's adjuvant-induced T cells prevent the development and adoptive transfer of diabetes in nonobese diabetic mice. *J Immunol.* 1993;150:2072–2080.

26. Kodama S, Kuhtreiber W, Fujimura S, Dale EA, Faustman DL. Islet regeneration during the reversal of autoimmune diabetes in NOD mice. *Science.* 2003;302:1223–1227.

27. Shehadeh N, Etzioni A, Cahana A, et al. Repeated BCG vaccination is more effective than a single dose in preventing diabetes in non-obese diabetic (NOD) mice. *Isr J Med Sci.* 1997;33:711–715.

28. Yang XD, Tisch R, Singer SM, et al. Effect of tumor necrosis factor alpha on insulin-dependent diabetes mellitus in NOD mice. I. The early development of autoimmunity and the diabetogenic process. *J Exp Med.* 1994;180:995–1004.

29. Tian B, Hao J, Zhang Y, et al. Upregulating CD4+CD25+FOXP3+ regulatory T cells in pancreatic lymph nodes in diabetic NOD mice by adjuvant immunotherapy. *Transplantation.* 2009;87:198–206.

30. Wu AJ, Hua H, Munson SH, McDevitt HO. Tumor necrosis factor-alpha regulation of CD4+CD25+ T cell levels in NOD mice. *Proc Natl Acad Sci USA.* 2002;99:12287–12292.

31. Ristori G, Romano S, Cannoni S, et al. Effects of Bacille Calmette-Guerin after the first demyelinating event in the CNS. *Neurology.* 2014;82:41–48.

32. Ristori G, Buzzi MG, Sabatini U, et al. Use of Bacille Calmette-Guerin (BCG) in multiple sclerosis. *Neurology.* 1999;53:1588–1589.

33. Paolillo A, Buzzi MG, Giugni E, et al. The effect of Bacille Calmette-Guerin on the evolution of new enhancing lesions to hypointense T1 lesions in relapsing remitting MS. *J Neurol.* 2003;250:247–248.

34. Ristori G, Romano S, Cannoni S, et al. Effects of the Bacillus Calmette-Guerin (BCG) vaccine in the demyelinating disease of the central nervous system. In: Faustman DL, ed. *The Value of BCG and TNF in Autoimmunity*. Boston, MA: Academic Press; 2014:63–80.
35. Shehadeh N, Calcinaro F, Bradley BJ, Bruchlim I, Vardi P, Lafferty KJ. Effect of adjuvant therapy on development of diabetes in mouse and man. *Lancet*. 1994;343:706–707.
36. Pozzilli P. BCG vaccine in insulin-dependent diabetes mellitus. IMDIAB Group. *Lancet*. 1997;349:1520–1521.
37. Allen HF, Klingensmith GJ, Jensen P, Simoes E, Hayward A, Chase HP. Effect of bacillus Calmette-Guerin vaccination on new-onset type 1 diabetes. A randomized clinical study. *Diabetes Care*. 1999;22:1703–1707.
38. Elliott JF, Marlin KL, Couch RM. Effect of bacille Calmette-Guerin vaccination on C-peptide secretion in children newly diagnosed with IDDM. *Diabetes Care*. 1998;21:1691–1693.
39. Hayashi D, Takii T, Fujiwara N, et al. Comparable studies of immunostimulating activities in vitro among Mycobacterium bovis bacillus Calmette-Guerin (BCG) substrains. *FEMS Immunol Med Microbiol*. 2009;56:116–128.
40. Ritz N, Hanekom WA, Robins-Browne R, Britton WJ, Curtis N. Influence of BCG vaccine strain on the immune response and protection against tuberculosis. *FEMS Microbiol Rev*. 2008;32:821–841.
41. Kuhtreiber WM, Leung SL, Wang L, et al. Possible transient benefits of Epstein Barr virus infection in three subjects with established type 1 diabetes. *J Diabetes Metab*. 2013;4:1000309.
42. Olleros ML, Guler R, Corazza N, et al. Transmembrane TNF induces an efficient cell-mediated immunity and resistance to *Mycobacterium bovis* Bacillus Calmette-Guérin infection in the absence of secreted TNF and lymphotoxin-α. *J Immunol*. 2002;168:3394–3401.
43. Okubo Y, Torrey H, Butterworth J, Zheng H, Faustman DL. Treg activation defect in type 1 diabetes: correction with TNFR2 agonism. *Clin Transl Immunol*. 2016;5:e56.
44. Chopra M, Biehl M, Steinfatt T, et al. Exogenous TNFR2 activation protects from acute GvHD via host T reg cell expansion. *J Exp Med*. 2016;213:1881–1900.
45. McGovern JL, Nguyen DX, Notley CA, Mauri C, Isenberg DA, Ehrenstein MR. Th17 cells are restrained by Treg cells via the inhibition of interleukin-6 in patients with rheumatoid arthritis responding to anti-tumor necrosis factor antibody therapy. *Arthritis Rheum*. 2012;64:3129–3138.
46. Grinberg-Bleyer Y, Saadoun D, Baeyens A, et al. Pathogenic T cells have a paradoxical protective effect in murine autoimmune diabetes by boosting Tregs. *J Clin Investig*. 2010;120:4558–4568.
47. Kleijwegt FS, Laban S, Duinkerken G, et al. Critical role for TNF in the induction of human antigen-specific regulatory T cells by tolerogenic dendritic cells. *J Immunol*. 2010;185:1412–1418.
48. Chopra M, Riedel SS, Biehl M, et al. Tumor necrosis factor receptor 2-dependent homeostasis of regulatory T cells as a player in TNF-induced experimental metastasis. *Carcinogenesis*. 2013;34:1296–1303.
49. Zaragoza B, Chen X, Oppenheim JJ, et al. Suppressive activity of human regulatory T cells is maintained in the presence of TNF. *Nat Med*. 2016;22:16–17.
50. Nguyen DX, Ehrenstein MR. Anti-TNF drives regulatory T cell expansion by paradoxically promoting membrane TNF-TNF-RII binding in rheumatoid arthritis. *J Exp Med*. 2016;213:1241–1253.
51. Punit S, Dube PE, Liu CY, Girish N, Washington MK, Polk DB. Tumor necrosis factor receptor 2 restricts the pathogenicity of CD8(+) T cells in mice with colitis. *Gastroenterology*. 2015;149:993–1005. e1002.

52. He X, Landman S, Bauland S, van den Dolder J, Koenen H, Joosten I. A TNFR2 agonist facilitates high purity expansion of human low purity Treg cells. *PloS One*. 2016;https://doi.org/10.1371/journal.pone.0156311.
53. Kühtreiber WM, Tran L, Taesoo K, Dybala M, Nguyen B, Plager S, Huang D, Janes S, Defusco S, Baum B, Zheng H, Faustman DL. Long-term reduction in hyperglycemia in advanced type 1 diabetes: the value of induced aerobic glycolysis with BCG vaccinations. Nature Vaccines June 23rd publication.

CHAPTER 3

Bacille Calmette-Guérin (BCG) Vaccine in Neuroinflammation

Silvia Romano*, Michela Ferraldeschi†, Maria Chiara Buscarinu*, Arianna Fornasiero*, Roberta Reniè*, Emanuele Morena*, Carmela Romano*, Rosella Mechelli*, Nicola Vanacore‡, Marco Salvetti*, Giovanni Ristori*

*Center for Experimental Neurological Therapies S. Andrea Hospital-site, Neurosciences, Mental Health, and Sensory Organs (NESMOS) Department, "Sapienza" University of Rome, Rome, Italy
†Department of Neurology and Psychiatry, "Sapienza" University of Rome, Rome, Italy
‡National Centre of Epidemiology, National Institute of Health, Rome, Italy

Contents

BACILLE CALMETTE-GUERIN (BCG) AND OTHER VACCINES IN MULTIPLE SCLEROSIS (MS)

Historical evidence on the beneficial effects of mycobacterial vaccine or adjuvant therapy in experimental models of autoimmune diseases (including Experimental Allergic Encephalomyelitis [EAE])[1–3] pointed to several works presented during the 1990s, which reinforced the rationale for this approach in neuroinflammation: the predominant recognition of conserved regions of mycobacterial heat shock proteins in both MS patients and healthy subjects,[4] the resistance to EAE induction by preimmunization with diverse antigens (both nonself and auto-antigens),[5] and the immune deviation toward a T helper 1 cytokine profile in MS patients with a satisfactory response to interferon beta therapy.[6] All of these results led to the hypothesis that immune stimulation mimicking benign microbial exposure could improve neuroinflammation, prompting us to perform the first study with BCG vaccine in patients with relapsing-remitting MS.[7]

The Value of BCG and TNF in Autoimmunity
https://doi.org/10.1016/B978-0-12-814603-3.00003-3

We carried out a single crossover trial[8] in relapsing-remitting patients with initial MS, with a primary end-point based on gadolinium (Gd)-enhanced magnetic resonance imaging (MRI) of the brain. After a baseline clinical-MRI evaluation, patients were followed-up monthly with Gd-enhanced MRI of the brain for 6 months of run-in, and for 6 months after a single dose of BCG vaccine. The effects of BCG were assessed, comparing disease activity at MRI during the run-in and post-BCG period. No adverse event occurred except for local reaction to inoculation in two patients. The frequency of Gd-enhancing lesions was higher during the run-in than after BCG (1.36 vs. 0.66; $P = .008$ by Wilcoxon signed rank test, corresponding to a 51% reduction). The frequency of active lesions (Gd-enhanced lesions plus new and enlarging lesions in T2-weighted-T2W images) was 2.27 during the run-in vs. 0.98 after BCG ($P = .008$), corresponding to a 57% reduction (Table 3.1). Overall, disease activity at MRI proved to be significantly lower during the post-BCG period.

This study confirmed the safety of another vaccine in MS (previous work from others and our group had showed safety of influenza vaccines).[9,10] Moreover, our results somehow anticipated those from a large study by Confavreux et al.[11] that patients with at least one confirmed vaccination in

Table 3.1 MRI activity before and after Bacille Calmette-Guèrin (BCG) in 12 patients with relapsing-remitting MS

	Active lesion frequency		Gd-enhancing lesion frequency	
Patient[a]	Run-in	Post-BCG	Run-in	Post-BCG
1	2.60	0.33	0.83	0.16
2	0	0	0	0
3	0	0.16	0	0.16
4	3	0.66	0.16	0
5	0.83	0.83	0.33	0.16
6	1.50	1	1	0.50
7	0.83	0.33	0.50	0.33
8	0.16	0	0	0
9	2.16	0.33	1.16	0.16
10	9.66	3.50	6.83	2.33
11	1	0.66	0.50	0.33
12	5.6	4	5	3.80
Median	1.25	0.49	0.5	0.16
Mean ± SE	2.27 ± 0.8	0.98 ± 0.4[b]	1.36 ± 0.6	0.66 ± 0.3[b]

[a] Two patients dropped out (pregnancy and shift to a very progressive form of disease during run-in); as these patients did not receive BCG vaccine, they were excluded from the analysis.
[b] $P = .008$ by Wilcoxon signed-rank test.

the observation period seemed to do significantly better in terms of both disability and the number of relapses than nonvaccinated controls (this difference was not related to other baseline characteristics of the patients studied). This study supported not only the safety but also the possible benefit of exposure to microbial products in MS, in the absence of infection as in the case of vaccinations.[12]

TEMPORAL DYNAMICS OF BCG VACCINE EFFECTS IN MS

In the same cohort of MS patients who participated in the crossover trial, we evaluated the effect of BCG vaccine on the evolution of new Gd-enhancing lesions to hypointense lesions on T1-weighted MRI images.[13] This allowed us to quantify the so-called black holes (BH), an expression of tissue damage, with the aim of evaluating vaccine influence on tissue damage, a crucial component of MS pathophysiology that underlies the development of clinical disability.[14–16] The percentage of new enhancing lesions (NEL) that evolve into BH is a measure of tissue damage that may result either from the severity of the inflammatory process or from primary axonal damage.

Patients who had participated in the single crossover trial underwent further MRI scans every 6 months for a total period of 24 months after vaccination. None of these patients took disease-modifying therapies (DMT) during the study period. We compared the outcome of NEL between the two phases of the trial: the run–in vs. the post-BCG percentage of NEL that evolved into BH. Table 3.2 summarize the results; a significant reduction of NEL was observed after BCG vaccine (58 vs. 28; $P < .01$ with χ^2 test) confirming the previous effect on disease activity at MRI. Gd-enhancement persisted at subsequent scans in 18 of the 58 (31%) NEL of the run–in phase and in 1 of the 28 (4%) NEL of the post-BCG phase ($P < .01$ by χ^2); the number of NEL evolving to BH was 28 of the 58 (46%) for those of

Table 3.2 Number and outcome of new enhancing lesions (NEL) at brain MRI

	Run-in phase	Post-BCG
Number of NEL	58	28[a]
Evolution to black holes at 24-month scan	28/58 (46%)	6/28 (21%)[a]
Persistence at subsequent MRI scan	18/58 (31%)	1/28 (4%)[a]

[a]$P \le .01$ with the χ^2 test.

the run-in phase and 6 of the 28 (21%) for those of the post–BCG period ($P < .01$ by χ^2).

This post hoc analysis seemed to indicate that vaccination with BCG might decrease tissue damage; the significantly lower persistence of NEL at subsequent MRI scans after BCG suggested that the decrease of duration (besides the frequency) of the inflammatory lesions might favor repair mechanisms. Moreover, the dynamics of BCG effects over time prompted us to hypothesize its long-term benefit and to design future studies on a longer temporal scale. The appropriate condition seemed to be the first demyelinating episode [usually referred to as clinically isolated syndrome (CIS)] considered to be the onset of clinical disease in the presence of a brain and spinal cord MRI compatible with MS, which had already been studied for the effects of interferon beta-1a over time at the end of the 1990s.[17]

BCG VACCINE IN CLINICALLY ISOLATED SYNDROMES (CIS)

Approximately half of people with CIS present with a new demyelinating episode converting to clinically definite MS (CDMS) within 2 years of diagnosis, whereas about 10% of CIS people remain free of further neurological events, even in the presence of a brain and spinal cord MRI compatible with MS.[18,19] For patients who convert, the risk of later progression of disability is substantial.[18–21] This justifies the administration of DMT usually indicated for MS in CIS subjects.[17,22,23]

Considering our previous encouraging results in patients with early MS,[7,13] and because it's a cheap, safe, and handy adjuvant approach, we considered BCG appropriate for people with CIS. We designed a trial based on the usual protocol for vaccination against *Mycobacterium tuberculosis*.[24] Participants were randomly assigned to receive either BCG vaccine or placebo, and were monitored monthly with brain MRI scans for 6 months. All individuals then entered a preplanned follow-up phase with intramuscular interferon beta-1a for another 12 months. Finally, an open-label extension was planned for up to 60 months after vaccine or placebo (from month 18 onward, patients were treated with the DMT that the neurologist in charge considered indicated) to evaluate long-term effects of BCG.

Seventy-three individuals with a first clinical event suggestive of MS were enrolled from three Italian MS centers. Demographic, clinical, and MRI characteristics were comparable between the two groups at baseline. Disease activity was reduced in the treated group during the 6-month follow-up (Table 3.3). No adverse event occurred after 6 months except for local reaction to inoculation in three subjects who were vaccinated.

The mean change in the number of total T1-hypointense lesions from the baseline to months 6, 12, and 18 showed virtually no accumulation in vaccinated CIS people, compared with an increased load in those receiving placebo: -0.09 ± 0.72 vs. 0.75 ± 1.81 ($P = .01$); 0.0 ± 0.83 vs. 0.88 ± 2.21 ($P = .08$); and -0.21 ± 1.03 vs. 1.00 ± 2.49 ($P = .02$), respectively, for each time point. After 18 months, the cumulative number of relapses was 25 of 40 (62.5%) in the placebo group vs. 10 of 33 (30.3%) in the BCG group (risk difference 32.2%, 95%CI 10.5%–53.9%; $P = .01$).

During follow-up at 5 years, we observed a significant difference between the BCG + DMT and placebo + DMT groups in the occurrence of the second demyelinating event (that is, conversion to CDMS). At the end of follow-up, more than half of vaccinated individuals remained relapse-free (19/33; 57.6%) compared with 12 of 40 (30%) in the placebo group, with an absolute difference of 27.6% ($P = .018$). A log rank test showed a different pattern of cumulative probability of CDMS in the two groups ($P = .02$). A Cox regression model adjusted for baseline data showed that the 5-years cumulative probability of CDMS was lower in the BCG + DMT group

Table 3.3 Disease activity at MRI and T1-hypointense lesions after 6 monthly scans following vaccination or placebo

Number	BCG $n = 33$	Placebo $n = 40$	RR[a] (95% CI) P value
New and enlarging T2-hyperintense lesions			
Mean ± SD	3.21±5.40	7.67 ± 12.66	0.364
Median (IQR)	1 (0–3)	2 (0.25–8.5)	(0.207–0.639)
Range	(0–20)	(0–49)	0.001
Total Gd-enhancing lesions			
Mean ± SD	3.09 ± 5.40	6.62 ± 11.84	0.541
Median (IQR)	0(0–2.5)	2 (0.25–6.0)	(0.308–0.956)
Range	(0–20)	(0–53)	0.033
New T1-hypointense lesions			
Mean ± SD	0.18±0.58	0.90 ± 1.93	0.149
Median (IQR)	0 (0–0)	0 (0–1)	(0.046–0.416)
Range	(0–3)	(0–10)	0.001

Abbreviation: *BCG*, Bacille Calmette-Guerin; *RR*, relative risk; *IQR*, interquartile range.
[a]Relative risk adjusted for baseline covariates (age, sex, EDSS, Gd-enhancing lesions, T2-hyperintense lesions, T1-hypointense lesions, clinical form at onset).

(HR = 0.52, 95%CI 0.27–0.99; P < .05). The mean time free of relapse was 42.94 ± 21.99 months in the BCG group vs. 32.45 ± 23.29 months in the placebo group (P < .05). No major adverse events were recorded during the trial. During follow-up, the frequency and nature of adverse events were within the established profile of DMT that the patients took, without any differences between vaccinated and nonvaccinated individuals.

This study extended the beneficial action of BCG vaccination to CIS people and confirmed the long-term potential of such an effect. In particular, the dynamics of the BH in our study suggest that a single vaccination with BCG may exert a plausibly long-lasting protective effect on tissue damage. Subsequent studies tried other DMT to prevent conversion to CDMS; besides interferon,[17] glatiramer acetate proved to be effective as well.[23] Among other more recent DMT, cladribine and teriflunomide proved to be effective,[25,26] whereas minocycline gave nonconclusive results.[27] Currently, BCG vaccine remains by far the handiest approach known to be effective in contributing to delaying conversion of CIS people to CDMS.

BCG VACCINE IN RADIOLOGICALLY ISOLATED SYNDROMES (RIS)

Following the extraordinary progress in the treatment of relapsing-remitting (RR) MS, two major unmet needs remain to be addressed by translational research in this field: progressive MS and the "dream" of a world free of MS. As far as the latter is concerned, we can hope to make the dream come true by understanding the etiology of the disease and therefore design definitive cures. Unfortunately, this perspective is neither at hand, nor can it be taken for granted that the etiologic targets, once discovered, will be readily treatable. A more realistic and pragmatic perspective may be the prevention of the clinical onset of the disease, a research field that promises to become increasingly important as the integration of genetic data with endophenotypes, MRI, and other biomarkers ameliorates our ability to predict the development of the disease under clinical circumstances.

Epidemiological data supporting vitamin D supplementation and smoking avoidance are candidate approaches for primary and secondary prevention of the disease. Among other interventions that may have characteristics compatible with those of a preventive treatment, BCG vaccine, which gave encouraging results in early MS[7,13] and CIS,[24] seems a suitable candidate. The knowledge that disease-modifying therapies work best when used early in the demyelinating process suggests the potential effectiveness of this handy approach in individuals with RIS.

RIS is a new entity, diagnosed when the unanticipated MRI finding of brain spatial dissemination of focal white matter (WM) lesions highly suggestive of MS occurs in subjects without symptoms of MS, and with normal neurological examinations.[28] Approximately one-third and two-thirds of individuals experience clinical onset and/or radiological progression, respectively, over a mean follow-up of 5 years. However, predictors (male sex, age < 37, spinal cord involvement) of higher risk of progression have been identified, and conversion to clinically isolated syndromes (CIS) were described in 84% of RIS individuals with spinal cord lesions over a median time of 1.6 years from the date of the first MRI. The same predictors have recently been shown to precede evolution toward primary progressive MS.[29–32] Whether or not to treat this condition currently remains a clinical conundrum.

Reasoning that an approach such as BCG vaccine seems appropriate as a frontline immunomodulatory approach for RIS people, we designed a 3-year longitudinal study project that takes into account the relative rarity of the RIS condition, as well as the need of an adequate follow-up to obtain informative outcome measures. We plan to vaccinate individuals with RIS, evaluating the impact of BCG by neuroimaging and immune-metabolic profiling. We considered an extension of the adjuvant approach to subjects with RIS timely, also considering recent achievements in "metrics" suitable to analyze this condition. Neuroimaging has recently allowed improvement of the characterization of RIS, including the identification of individuals at higher risk of progression to MS,[33] and disclosure of cortical lesions and axonal damage in the RIS brain.[34,35] Immune-metabolic profiling provides a complex correlation between immune and metabolic cellular variables,[36,37] which seem especially apt to analyze preclinical phases of neuroinflammation, and to study an approach whose underlying mechanisms of action remain largely unknown, in spite of encouraging clinical results.

We will randomize 100 persons with RIS according to Okuda criteria:[28] 50 will receive a single dose of BCG, and 50 will receive a single dose of placebo. The two groups will undergo the following procedures at baseline and at different time points (Table 3.4):

- Clinical status, including MS functional composite scale and symbol digit modality test, every 6 months for the 3-year follow-up.
- MRI brain scan at months 6, 12, 24, and 36.
- Immune-metabolic profiling, as recently described by Matarese's group,[36,37] at months 6, 12, 24, and 36.

The primary endpoint of the study will be the number of active T2 lesions developed over 1 year. The secondary endpoint will be the time to

Table 3.4 Flowchart

Activity	Visit 1 Day −2 → Day 1 Baseline Randomization treatment	Visit 2 6 months Follow-up visit	Visit 3 12 months Follow-up visit	Visit 4 24 months Follow-up visit	Visit 5 36 months End of study
Informed consent	x				
Inclusion/exclusion criteria	x				
Demographic data	x				
Medical history	x				
Concomitant medications	x	x	x	x	x
Physical examination	x	x	x	x	x
Neurological examination	x	x	x	x	x
Multiple sclerosis functional composite scale	x	x	x	x	x
Symbol digit modality test	x	x	x	x	x
Hematology and blood chemistry[a]	x	x	x	x	x
Urine examination	x				
Screening autoantibody and HIV serodiagnosis[b]	x				
Electrocardiogram	x				
X-ray chest	x				
Mantoux reaction	x				
Brain MRI scan	x	x	x	x	x
Immune metabolic profiling	x	x	x	x	x
Randomization	x				
Study drug/placebo injection distribute delivery to subject	x				
Adverse events	x	x	x	x	x

[a] Routine exams (ESR, CBC, GOT, GPT, gamma GT, total bilirubin, coagulation, creatinine, BUN, glucose, serum protein electrophoresis) and pregnancy test for female (only at screening).
[b] Screening autoantibody: antinuclear antibodies (ANA) anti-DNA antibodies, etc.

the first clinical event over the 3-year period. Exploratory MRI-based endpoints (cortical lesions, brain volume changes, and magnetization transfer ratios) will be also considered for the 3-year follow-up. A multiple parameter analysis will be applied to monitor changes in the immune-metabolic profiling before and after BCG. Safety and feasibility of this approach will be assessed. The clinical progression (that is, the conversion to CIS) will determine the exit of the subject from the blind procedure (when possible, an unblinded follow-up to 36 months from vaccine or placebo will continue with the same methods as the RIS subjects).

BCG VACCINE IN NEUROINFLAMMATION AND NEURODEGENERATIVE DISEASES

Recent evidence consistently showed a neuroinflammatory component in common neurodegenerative diseases, such as Alzheimer's disease (AD) and Parkinson's disease (PD), with a prevalent role for glial cells and innate immune systems.[38] A neuroinflammatory response involving polarized microglial activity, enhanced astrocyte reactivity, and elevated proinflammatory cytokine and chemokine load in the brain has been proposed to facilitate neurodegeneration.[39] In this context, several papers reported a neuroprotective action of BCG vaccine in experimental models of neurodegenerative diseases and neurodevelopment disorders. Two works in models of PD suggested a BCG-mediated immune stimulation that may limit deleterious microglial response to a neuronal insult,[40] and may promote T regulatory protective responses.[41] Two other works in models of AD elucidated additional mechanisms of neuroprotection: activation of tumor necrosis factor receptor 2 (TNFR2) that blocks neuroinflammation and promotes neuronal survival,[42] as well as recruitment of inflammation-resolving monocyte (producing antiinflammatory cytokines and neurotrophic factors) at the choroid plexus and perivascular spaces of plaque pathology.[43] Along the same line of research, several works showed a beneficial effect of neonatal BCG vaccination on neurodevelopment. In one study, it proved to reinforce the cognitive skills via a shift in meningeal macrophage M2 polarization and neurotrophic factor expression.[44] Another work reported BCG vaccination ameliorated neurobehavioral impairment and neuroinflammation (sickness, anxiety, and depression-like behavior; impairment in hippocampal cell proliferation; and proinflammatory responses in serum and brain) due to secondary immune challenge in adult mice.[45]

All these data coming from recent works in neurodegenerative diseases, including beneficial, long-lasting action of neonatal BCG vaccination, are reminiscent of a robust corpus of evidence that have been growing for decades in inflammatory (sensu stricto) and immune-mediated conditions. Recently defined "trained immunity" has been extensively studied in BCG-vaccinated subjects relating to beneficial, nonspecific (or heterologous) effects ranging from protection against nonmycobacterial infective diseases, decreased incidence of allergic diseases, immune-modulatory effects in autoimmune disorders, and treatment of certain malignancies.[46,47] Trained immunity seems to be prevalently mediated by cells of the innate immunity, whereby epigenetic, long-lasting mechanisms impact on immunometabolic pathways and exert effects on heterologous adaptive immune responses.[48–50] Trained immunity is part of a virtuous circle, apparently triggered by BCG vaccination, that has been elucidated in several studies on type 1 diabetes and MS, including their experimental models,[7,13,24,51–55] as well as on childhood infection.[56,57]

This virtuous circle include apoptosis of pathogenic clonotypic cells, induction of regulatory T cells and antiinflammatory monocytes, and fostering of tissue repair, especially through agonistic action on TNFR2[58,59] (Fig. 3.1). In particular, the role of BCG vaccine as a TNF-inducer seems very important to mediate its beneficial effects on immune modulation and tissue repair; TNFR2 activation was recently reported to mediate expansion of T regulatory cells and myeloid-derived suppressor cell in different contexts, such as graft versus host disease and tumor microenvironment.[60,61]

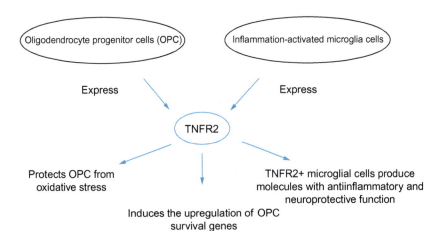

Fig. 3.1 Role of TNRF2 receptor in neuroinflammation. *(From Veroni C, Gabriele L, Canini I, Castiello L, Coccia E, Remoli ME, et al. Activation of TNF receptor 2 in microglia promotes induction of anti-inflammatory pathways. Mol Cell Neurosci. 2010;45(3):234–44; Maier O, Fischer R, Agresti C, Pfizenmaier K. TNF receptor 2 protects oligodendrocyte progenitor cells against oxidative stress. Biochem Biophys Res Commun. 2013;440(2):336–41.)*

Overall, it seems that BCG vaccination might trigger mechanisms that mediate immunoregulation and immune training at the same time, along with tissue repair, in diverse pathological conditions that share chronic inflammation and tissue damage. Protection against these shared contexts may, at least in part, be explained by the "old friends" hypothesis[62] (that resumes and somehow overcomes the "hygiene" hypothesis). It postulates that a deprivation of exposure to immunoregulatory, environmental microorganisms may determine a chronic, low-level inflammation that poses a risk for many, highly prevalent, diseases in developed countries. BCG vaccination might somehow compensate for this deprivation and restore an exposure to one of the most ancient "old friends," with which human beings coevolved and coexpanded since the out-of-Africa migration and Neolithic age.[63]

REFERENCES

1. Kies MW, Alvord Jr. EC. Prevention of allergic encephalomyelitis by prior injection of adjuvants. *Nature*. 1958;182(4642):1106.
2. Hempel K, Freitag A, Freitag B, Endres B, Mai B, Liebaldt G. Unresponsiveness to experimental allergic encephalomyelitis in Lewis rats pretreated with complete Freund's adjuvant. *Int Arch Allergy Appl Immunol*. 1985;76(3):193–199.
3. Singh B. Stimulation of the developing immune system can prevent autoimmunity. *J Autoimmun*. 1990;14:15–22.
4. Salvetti M, Ristori G, Buttinelli C, et al. The immune response to mycobacterial 70-kDa heat shock proteins frequently involves autoreactive T cells and is quantitatively disregulated in multiple sclerosis. *J Neuroimmunol*. 1996;65(2):143–153.
5. Fiori P, Ristori G, Cacciani A, et al. Down-regulation of cell-surface CD4 co-receptor expression and modulation of experimental allergic encephalomyelitis. *Int Immunol*. 1997;9(4):541–545.
6. Ristori G, Montesperelli C, Gasperini C, et al. T cell response to myelin basic protein before and after treatment with interferon beta in multiple sclerosis. *J Neuroimmunol*. 1999;99(1):91–96.
7. Ristori G, Buzzi MG, Sabatini U, et al. Use of Bacille Calmette-Guèrin (BCG) in multiple sclerosis. *Neurology*. 1999;53:1588–1589.
8. McFarland HF, Frank JA, Albert PS, et al. Using gadolinium-enhanced magnetic resonance imaging lesions to monitor disease activity in multiple sclerosis. *Ann Neurol*. 1992;32:758–766.
9. Salvetti M, Pisani A, Bastianello S, Millefiorini E, Buttinelli C, Pozzilli C. Clinical and MRI assessment of disease activity in patients with multiple sclerosis after influenza vaccination. *J Neurol*. 1995;242:143–146.
10. Miller AE, Morgante LA, Buchwald LY, et al. A multicenter, randomized, double-blind, placebo-controlled trial of influenza immunization in multiple sclerosis. *Neurology*. 1997;48:312–314.
11. Confavreux C, Suissa S, Saddier P, Bourdès V, Vukusic S. Vaccines in multiple sclerosis study group. Vaccinations and the risk of relapse in multiple sclerosis. *N Engl J Med*. 2001;344(5):319–326.
12. Buttinelli C, Salvetti M, Ristori G. Vaccination and the risk of relapse in multiple sclerosis. *N Engl J Med*. 2001;344:1794.

13. Paolillo A, Buzzi MG, Giugni E, et al. The effect of Bacille Calmette-Guerin on the evolution of the new enhancing lesions to hypointense T1 lesions in relapsing-remitting MS. *J Neurol.* 2003;250:247–248.
14. van Waesberghe JH, Kamphorst W, De Groot CJ, et al. Axonal loss in multiple sclerosis lesions: magnetic resonance imaging insights into substrates of disability. *Ann Neurol.* 1999;46:747–754.
15. van Walderveen MA, Barkhof F, Pouwels PJ, van Schijndel RA, Polman CH, Castelijns JA. Neuronal damage in T1-hypointense multiple sclerosis lesions demonstrated in vivo using proton magnetic resonance spectroscopy. *Ann Neurol.* 1999;46:79–87.
16. Brex PA, Parker GJ, Leary SM, Molyneux PD, Barker GJ, Davie CA. Lesion heterogeneity in MS: a study of the relationships between appearance on T1-weighted images, T1 relaxation times and metabolite concentrations. *J Neurol Neurosurg Psychiatry.* 2000;68:627–632.
17. Jacobs LD, Beck RW, Simon JH, et al. Intramuscular interferon beta-1a therapy initiated during a first demyelinating event in multiple sclerosis. CHAMPS study group. *N Engl J Med.* 2000;343:898–904.
18. Brex PA, Ciccarelli O, O'Riordan JI, Sailer M, Thompson AJ, Miller DH. A longitudinal study of abnormalities on MRI and disability from multiple sclerosis. *N Engl J Med.* 2002;346:158–164.
19. Miller D, Barkhof F, Montalban X, Thompson A, Filippi M. Clinically isolated syndromes suggestive of multiple sclerosis, part I: natural history, pathogenesis, diagnosis, and prognosis. *Lancet Neurol.* 2005;4:281–288.
20. Tintoré M, Rovira A, Río J, et al. Baseline MRI predicts future attacks and disability in clinically isolated syndromes. *Neurology.* 2006;67:968–972.
21. Fisniku LK, Brex PA, Altmann DR, et al. Disability and T2 MRI lesions: a 20-year follow-up of patients with relapse onset of multiple sclerosis. *Brain.* 2008;131:808–817.
22. Comi G, Filippi M, Barkhof F, et al, the Early treatment of Multiple Sclerosis Study Group. Effect of early interferon treatment on conversion to definite multiple sclerosis: a randomised study. *Lancet.* 2001;357:1576–1582.
23. Comi G, Martinelli V, Rodegher M, et al. Effect of glatiramer acetate on conversion to clinically definite multiple sclerosis in patients with clinically isolated syndrome (PreCISe study): a randomized, double-blind, placebo-controlled trial. *Lancet.* 2009;374:1503–1511.
24. Ristori G, Romano S, Cannoni S, et al. Effects of Bacille Calmette-Guerin after the first demyelinating event in the CNS. *Neurology.* 2014;82(1):41–48.
25. Leist TP, Comi G, Cree BA, et al, Oral cladribine for early MS (ORACLE MS) Study Group. Effect of oral cladribine on time to conversion to clinically definite multiple sclerosis in patients with a first demyelinating event (ORACLE MS): a phase 3 randomised trial. *Lancet Neurol.* 2014;13(3):257–267.
26. Miller AE, Wolinsky JS, Kappos L, et al, TOPIC Study Group. Oral teriflunomide for patients with a first clinical episode suggestive of multiple sclerosis (TOPIC): a randomised, double-blind, placebo-controlled, phase 3 trial. *Lancet Neurol.* 2014;13(10):977–986.
27. Metz LM, Li DKB, Traboulsee AL, et al, Minocycline in MS Study Team. Trial of minocycline in a clinically isolated syndrome of multiple sclerosis. *N Engl J Med.* 2017;376(22):2122–2133.
28. Okuda DT, Mowry EM, Beheshtian A, et al. Incidental MRI anomalies suggestive of multiple sclerosis: the radiologically isolated syndrome. *Neurology.* 2009;72(9):800–805.
29. Granberg T, Martola J, Kristoffersen-Wiberg M, Aspelin P, Fredrikson S. Radiologically isolated syndrome-incidental magnetic resonance imaging findings suggestive of multiple sclerosis, a systematic review. *Mult Scler.* 2013;19(3):271–280.
30. Okuda DT, Siva A, Kantarci O, et al. Radiologically isolated syndrome: 5-year risk for an initial clinical event. *PLoS One.* 2014;9(3):e90509.

31. Okuda DT, Mowry EM, Cree BA, et al. Asymptomatic spinal cord lesions predict disease progression in radiologically isolated syndrome. *Neurology*. 2011;76(8):686–692.
32. Kantarci OH, Lebrun C, Siva A, et al. Primary progressive MS evolving from radiologically isolated syndrome. *Ann Neurol*. 2016;79(2):288–294.
33. De Stefano N, Stromillo ML, Rossi F, et al. Improving the characterization of radiologically isolated syndrome suggestive of multiple sclerosis. *PLoS One*. 2011;6(4):e19452.
34. Stromillo ML, Giorgio A, Rossi F, et al. Brain metabolic changes suggestive of axonal damage in radiologically isolated syndrome. *Neurology*. 2013;80(23):2090–2094.
35. Giorgio A, Stromillo ML, Rossi F, et al. Cortical lesions in radiologically isolated syndrome. *Neurology*. 2011;77(21):1896–1899.
36. Galgani M, Nugnes R, Bruzzese D, et al. Meta-immunological profiling of children with type 1 diabetes identifies new biomarkers to monitor disease progression. *Diabetes*. 2013;62(7):2481–2491.
37. Carbone F, De Rosa V, Carrieri PB, et al. Regulatory T cell proliferative potential is impaired in human autoimmune disease. *Nat Med*. 2013;20(1):69–74.
38. Ransohoff RM. How neuroinflammation contributes to neurodegeneration. *Science*. 2016;353(6301):777–783.
39. Minter MR, Taylor JM, Crack PJ. The contribution of neuroinflammation to amyloid toxicity in Alzheimer's disease. *J Neurochem*. 2016;136(3):457–474.
40. Yong J, Lacan G, Dang H, et al. BCG vaccine-induced neuroprotection in a mouse model of Parkinson's disease. *PLoS One*. 2011;6(1):e16610.
41. Laćan G, Dang H, Middleton B, et al. Bacillus Calmette-Guerin vaccine-mediated neuroprotection is associated with regulatory T-cell induction in the 1-methyl-4-phenyl-1,2,3,6-tetrahydropyridine mouse model of Parkinson's disease. *J Neurosci Res*. 2013;91(10):1292–1302.
42. Dong Y, Fischer R, Naudé PJ, et al. Essential protective role of tumor necrosis factor. Receptor 2 in neurodegeneration. *Proc Natl Acad Sci USA*. 2016;113(43):12304–12309.
43. Zuo Z, Qi F, Yang J, et al. Immunization with Bacillus Calmette-Guérin (BCG) alleviates neuroinflammation and cognitive deficits in APP/PS1 mice via the recruitment of inflammation-resolving monocytes to the brain. *Neurobiol Dis*. 2017;101:27–39.
44. Qi F, Zuo Z, Yang J, et al. Combined effect of BCG vaccination and enriched environment promote neurogenesis and spatial cognition via a shift in meningeal macrophage M2 polarization. *J Neuroinflammation*. 2017;14(1):32.
45. Yang J, Qi F, Yao Z. Neonatal BCG vaccianation alleviates lipopolysaccharide-induced neurobehavioral impairments and neuroinflammation in adult mice. *Mol Med Rep*. 2016;14(2):1574–1586.
46. Netea MG, van Crevel R. BCG-induced protection: effects on innate immune memory. *Semin Immunol*. 2014;26(6):512–517.
47. Töpfer E, Boraschi D, Italiani P. Innate immune memory: the latest frontier of adjuvanticity. *J Immunol Res*. 2015;2015:478408.
48. Kleinnijenhuis J, Quintin J, Preijers F, et al. Bacille Calmette-Guerin induces NOD2-dependent nonspecific protection from reinfection via epigenetic reprogramming of monocytes. *Proc Natl Acad Sci USA*. 2012;109(43):17537–17542.
49. Kleinnijenhuis J, Quintin J, Preijers F, et al. Long-lasting effects of BCG vaccination on both heterologous Th1/Th17 responses and innate trained immunity. *J Innate Immun*. 2014;6(2):152–158.
50. Arts RJ, Carvalho A, La Rocca C, et al. Immunometabolic pathways in BCG-induced trained immunity. *Cell Rep*. 2016;17(10):2562–2571.
51. Faustman D, Davis M. TNF receptor 2 pathways: drug target for autoimmune diseases. *Nat Rev Drug Discov*. 2010;9:482–493.

52. Faustman DL, Wang L, Okubo Y, et al. Proof-of-concept, randomized, controlled clinical trial of Bacillus-Calmette-Guerin for treatment of long-term type 1 diabetes. *PLoS One.* 2012;7(8):e41756.

53. Okubo Y, Mera T, Wang L, Faustman DL. Homogeneous expansion of human T-regulatory cells via tumor necrosis factor receptor 2. *Sci Rep.* 2013;3:3153.

54. Madsen PM, Motti D, Karmally S, et al. Oligodendroglial TNFR2 mediates membrane TNF-dependent repair in experimental autoimmune encephalomyelitis by promoting oligodendrocyte differentiation and remyelination. *J Neurosci.* 2016;36(18):5128–5143.

55. Gao H, Danzi MC, Choi CS, et al. Opposing functions of microglial and macrophagic TNFR2 in the pathogenesis of experimental autoimmune encephalomyelitis. *Cell Rep.* 2017;18(1):198–212.

56. De Castro MJ, Pardo-Seco J, Martinon-Torres F. Nonspecific (heterologous) protection of neonatal BCG vaccination against hospitalization due to respiratory infection and sepsis. *Clin Infect Dis.* 2015;60(11):1611–1619.

57. Kulkarni S, Mukherjee S, Pandey A, Dahake R, Padmanabhan U, Chowdhary AS. Bacillus Calmette-Guérin confers neuroprotection in a murine model of Japanese encephalitis. *Neuroimmunomodulation.* 2016;23(5–6):278–286.

58. Veroni C, Gabriele L, Canini I, et al. Activation of TNF receptor 2 in microglia promotes induction of anti-inflammatory pathways. *Mol Cell Neurosci.* 2010;45(3):234–244.

59. Maier O, Fischer R, Agresti C, Pfizenmaier K. TNF receptor 2 protects oligodendrocyte progenitor cells against oxidative stress. *Biochem Biophys Res Commun.* 2013;440(2):336–341.

60. Chopra M, Biehl M, Steinfatt T, et al. Exogenous TNFR2 activation protects from acute GvHD via host T reg cell expansion. *J Exp Med.* 2016;213(9):1881–1900.

61. Zhao X, Rong L, Zhao X, et al. TNF signaling drives myeloid-derived suppressor cell accumulation. *J Clin Invest.* 2012;122(11):4094–4104.

62. Reber SO, Siebler PH, Donner NC, et al. Immunization with a heat-killed preparation of the environmental bacterium Mycobacterium vaccae promotes stress resilience in mice. *Proc Natl Acad Sci USA.* 2016;113(22):E3130–9.

63. Comas I, Coscolla M, Luo T, et al. Out-of-Africa migration and Neolithic coexpansion of Mycobacterium tuberculosis with modern humans. *Nat Genet.* 2013;45(10):1176–1182.

CHAPTER 4

Host Epigenetic Modifications in *Mycobacterium tuberculosis* Infection: A Boon or Bane

Mona Singh*, **Vinod Yadav**†, **Gobardhan Das***
*Special Centre for Molecular Medicine, Jawaharlal Nehru University, New Delhi, India
†Department of Microbiology, Central University of Haryana, Mahendergarh, India

Contents

INTRODUCTION

The essence of epigenetics comes from the Greek word "epigenesis" meaning "in addition to genesis" or "above genetics." When Waddington coined this term in 1942, he described this as an additional mechanism of inheritance apart from standard genetics. Epigenetics helped many researchers to solve puzzles related to the functioning of gene(s) and suggested the possibility of alterations of gene(s) activity without changing the sequence.[1,2] Soon it became a popular avenue of research, and further discoveries reported that some of these epigenetic modifications are reversible. These modifications are also termed epigenetic tags, which maintain the dynamics between chromatin organization and cellular processes such as gene expression and recombination, DNA repair, etc. These epigenetic tags involve chromatin modification, DNA methylation, and RNA interference. A wide range of modifications, that is, methylation, acetylation, phosphorylation, ubiquitylation, and sumolyation, can modulate gene expression.[3–7]

The Value of BCG and TNF in Autoimmunity
https://doi.org/10.1016/B978-0-12-814603-3.00004-5
39

Most health indicators, behaviors, and a wide variety of diseases like cancer, autoimmune disease, respiratory illness, cognitive dysfunction, etc. are governed by epigenetics.[3] Several environmental factors, including environmental contaminants such as pesticides, heavy metals, tobacco smoke, polycyclic aromatic hydrocarbons (PAH), and radioactivity, along with other factors like microbes, nutrients, and hormones, are recognized as drivers of epigenetic modifications.[3] In recent years, pathogenic microbes have been reported as one of the crucial factors with the potential of epigenetic modulation of the host transcriptional program. This process acts by enforcing changes at the gene level, targeting different vital cellular processes such as immunity, apoptosis, and survival. It is well established that many successful human pathogens have evolved multiple mechanisms to escape host defense mechanisms.[8–13] They have the ability to reprogram the host genome to facilitate their survival within the host.[14] *Mycobacterium tuberculosis* (*M.tb*) is one classical example of those successful microorganisms that can modulate the host immune system for their survival.

M.tb, an obligate, aerobic bacteria, is the causative agent of tuberculosis (TB), responsible for approximately 2 million deaths every year.[15] Airborne particles called droplet nuclei of 1 to 5 μm in diameter are carriers of the pathogen, which is highly contagious.[16] A person with either pulmonary or laryngeal TB is the source of these droplet nuclei, which are produced through coughing, sneezing, and shouting. Most infections are asymptomatic, which is known as latent TB, where bacteria persist in a dormant condition. About 10% of latent TB cases progress to active disease in immune-compromised individuals. The widely accepted therapy for the treatment of TB, called Directly Observed Short Treatment Course (DOTS), involves the use of multiple antibiotics and is lengthy. Patients infected with drug-sensitive *M.tb* strains require a period of 6 months to complete treatment. The initial phase (2 months) involves treatment with Isoniazid, Rifampicin, Ethambutol, and Pyrazinamide, followed by treatment with Isoniazid and Rifampicin during the later phase (4 months).[17–19] However, therapeutic efficacy of these drugs is under serious consideration due to the emergence of multidrug-resistant TB (MDR-TB) and extensively drug-resistant TB (XDR-TB) strains.[20–24] MDR/XDR TB treatment is not only expensive but also involves exposure to toxic drugs for a period of almost 20 months with lower success rates. A WHO report estimated 4.5 lakhs MDR-TB cases every year, with 30% mortality and 10% of them further developing into XDR-TB.[15] In the current scenario, one-third

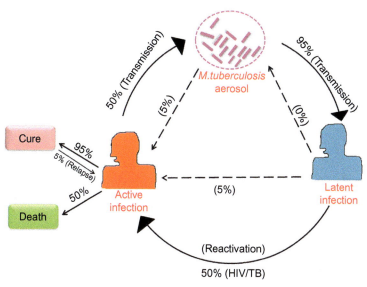

Fig. 4.1 Diagrammatic representation of the pathogenesis and latency of tuberculosis.

of the world population is infected with *M.tb*, whereas only ~10% are diagnosed for active TB. The fact that not all *M.tb*-infected individuals develop clinical disease needs serious consideration. Depending upon the state of the host immune system and the bacterial load, TB infection may become active or latent, or may be cleared from the system (Fig. 4.1).[25] Latent TB is merely detectable by standard diagnostic methods and can relapse as active TB in immune-compromised individuals. Taken together, the primary basis of TB infection depends upon the host immune system, which is further regulated by both internal and external factors such as nutrition, the environment, etc.[26]

In this chapter, we will describe the role of epigenetics in host immune evasion by *M.tb*. This chapter will deal with different epigenetic tags such as chromatin modifications, DNA methylation, and RNA interference that assists *M.tb* to modulate the host epigenome for its survival.

EPIGENETIC MODIFICATIONS: A MECHANISTIC APPROACH

Epigenetic modulation works mainly through three different way, that is, DNA methylation, histone modification, and noncoding RNA-mediated gene silencing.

DNA Methylation

Prior to 1980, multiple studies by McGhee & Ginder suggested that methylation has an important role in the regulation of gene expression.[27] DNA methylation represents a principle epigenetic tag in which a methyl group is attached to a cytosine residue at the C5 position (Fig. 4.2). This methylation tag is very common at CpG islands. The principle enzyme involved in this process is DNA methyltransferase (DNMTs). This enzyme exists in several isoforms known to play different functions. One of the isoforms, DNMT1, is the most abundant isoform and methylates unmethylated CpG residues, whereas the other isoform, DNMT3a/b, methylates both unmethylated and hemimethylated CpG islands. However, the rate of methylation is faster in the case of DNMT1.[28,29] Although epigenetic tags are mostly irreversible, DNA methylation can be reversed in DNA repair and during the DNA replication process.[30] DNA methylation can influence processes such as development, differentiation, reprogramming, and gene silencing, and can even modulate cancer cells.[31,32] CpG methylation silences gene expression either by recruiting corepressors or by preventing the association of DNA binding factors to their consensus binding sequences.[31,32] DNA methylation is known as the most stable epigenetic tag and thus can be responsible for long-term gene silencing (Fig. 4.2).

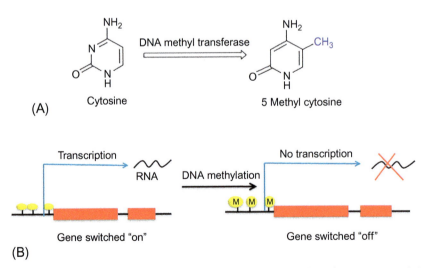

Fig. 4.2 (A) Methylation of cytosine. (B) DNA methylation mediated transcriptional silencing of gene promoters.

Histone Modifications

The genomic DNA in eukaryotic cells is packaged around special proteins termed histones to form protein/DNA complexes called chromatin.[33] The basic unit of chromatin is the nucleosome, which is composed of ~146 base pairs (bp) of DNA wrapped around an octamer of the four core histones (H2A, H2B, H3, and H4). The core histones are tightly packed in globular regions, with amino-terminal tails that extend from the globular region, making them accessible to histone-modifying enzymes. Another protein, termed linker histone H1, interacts with DNA and links two nucleosomes.[34,35] It functions in the compaction of chromatin into higher-order structures that comprise chromosomes. This organization of chromatin plays an important role in various nuclear processes like DNA replication, transcription, recombination, and DNA repair.[6,34] Chromatin can be divided into two functional states: euchromatin or heterochromatin, which are transcriptionally active or inactive states of chromatin, or areas of the chromosomes, respectively. Formation of euchromatin and heterochromatin is a dynamic process, tightly regulated by various remodeling and modifying mechanisms.[35,36] Euchromatin is the region where DNA is accessible, representing an open conformation due to the relaxed state of nucleosome arrangements. The genomic regions of euchromatin are more flexible and contain genes in active and inactive transcriptional states. Conversely, heterochromatin are areas where DNA is packaged into highly condensed forms inaccessible to transcription factors or chromatin-associated proteins. The genomic regions within heterochromatin primarily consist of repetitive sequences and repressed genes associated with morphogenesis or differentiation (imprinting or X chromosome inactivation). Altogether, chromatin structures regulate the outcome of various nuclear processes such as gene expression, silencing, DNA replication, transcription, recombination, DNA repair, and genome stability.[37–40]

Histone modification is a covalent posttranslational modification (PTM) of histone protein. The PTMs of histones can impact gene expression by altering chromatin structure or recruiting histone modifiers. The amino terminals of the core histone are subjected to several types of multivalent modifications, including acetylation, methylation, phosphorylation, ubiquitination, sumoylation, etc. Histone modifications are critical for regulating chromatin structure and function, which can in turn affect many DNA-related processes, such as transcription, recombination, repair and replication of DNA,[41–43] and chromosomal organization.[5] These histone modifications are categorized into eight different classes of posttranslational modification involving more than 60 distinct modification sites, namely lysine acetylation, ubiquitination and sumoylation, serine, threonine and tyrosine phosphory-lation, lysine and arginine methylation, glutamate poly-ADP ribosylation, arginine deamination, and proline isomerization, and altogether constitute the differences in dynamics and function of chromatin.[6,44] For instance, as-sociation of PTM at histone 3 lysine 4 residue trimethylation (H3K4me3) is related with active chromatin, whereas histone 3 lysine 9 residue trimeth-ylation (H3K9me3) is the characteristic of repressed chromatin.[45,46] These modifications are guided by different types of enzymes like kinases, histone methyltransferases (HMTs) and histone acetyltransferases (HATs), phospha-tases, histone demethylases (HDMs), and histone deacetylases (HDACs).[28,47,48] The acetylation of histones was the first epigenetic modification connected with biological activity. The lysine residues at the N-terminal of histone tails are subjected to either acetylation by histone acetyltransferase enzymes (HATs) or deacetylation by histone deacetylases (HDACs).[49,50]

The action of HATs acetylates histone tails, leading to an increase in space between nucleosomes and thus activates chromatin, whereas HDAC-mediated deacetylation suppresses the expression (Fig. 4.3).[40] In con-trast, histone methylation can either lead to transcriptional activation or

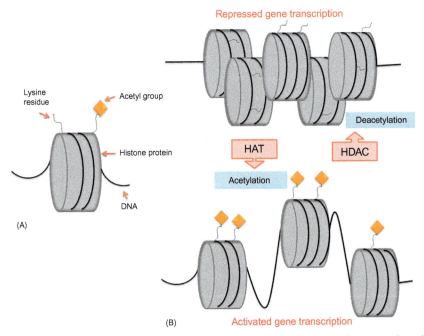

Fig. 4.3 (A) Structure of nucleosome. (B) DNA acetylation and deacetylation mediated activation and suppression of gene transcription.

inactivation of genomic regions.[6,41] It acts on different lysine residues and can add one, two, or three methyl groups. The impact of methylation not only depends on specific lysine residues but also on its degree of methylation. For example, transcriptional repression or heterochromatin formation can be mediated by H3K9me3, H3K27me3, and K4K20me3, whereas monomethylation at these residues, that is, H3K9me1, H3K27me1, and K4K20me1, can activate these genes.[45,46]

Altogether, these histones code control gene regulation and are very complex in nature. The outcome of gene activity depends on various other epigenetic factors that function synergistically with histones and thus determine the fate of gene transcription. Furthermore, it will be interesting to observe these epigenetic modifications within the host genome after infection with *M.tb.* The histone codes are so efficiently maintained that the same stimuli can induce the expression of a gene at one locus and can repress a gene at another locus. Therefore, it will be worthwhile to explore the mechanism by which these histone-modifying enzymes precisely modulate specific gene loci within the whole genome of the cell.

Noncoding RNAs

Based on in-silico approaches, the whole genome sequencing and transcriptomic analysis revealed that large numbers of transcribed RNAs are untranslated and thus predicted the existence of noncoding RNAs (ncRNAs). These ncRNAs play pivotal regulatory roles in various cellular functions. ncRNAs, also called microRNAs (miRNAs), were initially reported in 2001. Since then, they have been shown to constitute a large family of small ncRNAs. They can be further classified into several other forms including small nuclear RNAs (snRNAs), small interfering RNAs (siRNAs), small nucleolar RNAs (snoRNAs), and piwi-interacting RNAs (piRNAs). These miRNAs are highly conserved and function as endogenous gene silencers by repressing target mRNA at a translational level. They have been reported to be present in the genomes of animals, plants, and viruses. Studies have reported that miRNAs may play a role in regulating about 30% of all mammalian genes.[51–53] Their decisive roles in development, differentiation, apoptosis, and oncogenesis have been experimentally established.[54,55] The synthesis of miRNAs takes place in the nucleus as long primary transcripts (pri-miRNAs) and has imperfect hairpin structures. These are predominantly transcribed by RNA polymerase II (Pol II), although in some cases transcription can also be mediated by Pol III. Thereafter, with the help of RNase III, Drosha, and DGCR8, the pri-miRNAs is converted into

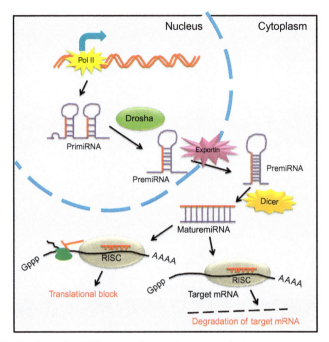

Fig. 4.4 Mechanism of miRNA processing and gene regulation.

precursor miRNA (pre-miRNA) molecules. Subsequently, the RNAse III Dicer enzyme cooperates with other factors and processes the pre-miRNAs into mature miRNAs as well as a complementary fragment called miRNA. Further, these mature miRNAs, along with the RNA-induced silencing complex (RISC), guides gene regulation processes[56–59] (Fig. 4.4). A number of studies have shown that miRNAs are involved in the regulation of important cellular pathways, such as apoptosis, cell proliferation, angiogenesis, and invasion, and in chromatin structure dynamics and genome organization in the nucleus, which has added additional complexity to epigenetic mechanisms.[60–62]

EPIGENETIC MODIFICATIONS: A TOOL EMPLOYED BY *M. TUBERCULOSIS* TO PROMOTE ITS SURVIVAL

M.tb has developed numerous mechanisms to hijack cellular processes to escape the host immune response. *M.tb* modulates the host both at genetic and epigenetic levels for its survival. These adaptations help *M.tb* to adapt to its environment inside host cells and promote its survival, growth, and latency. Both innate and adaptive immunity play important roles in combating *M.tb* infection.

ROLE OF CHROMATIN MODIFICATIONS IN *M.TB* INFECTION AND IMMUNE EVASION

Bacterial mechanisms of immune evasion involving control of gene expression at the chromatin level show high levels of complexity. Major histocompatibility complex (MHC) class II antigen presentation and subsequent CD4+ T-cell activation are critical for acquired immunity to *M.tb* infection. Studies have shown that IFN-γ generated by activated T cells and natural killer cells (NK cells) induce the surface expression of MHC class II in various cell types.[63] Further, the interaction of IFN-γ with its respective receptor activates the Janus tyrosine kinase-signal transducer and activator of transcription (JAK-STAT1) signaling cascade, which controls expression of several genes at the transcriptional level. This includes Class II major histocompatibility complex transactivator (CIITA), which plays a pivotal role in the transcription of genes associated with the MHC class II antigen-processing pathway.[64] However, one of the immune evasive mechanisms of *M.tb* includes inhibition of IFN-γ induced genes like CIITA, CD64, and HLA-DR through histone modification and chromatin remodeling at specific promoters.[65,66] Supression of CIITA transcription is mainly due to inhibition of SWI/SNF binding and histone deacetylation at the CIITA promoter, and conversely *M.tb* induces binding of the transcriptional repressor C/EBP to the CIITA promoter (Fig. 4.5).[67] Similarly, *M.tb*-infected cells inhibit HLA-DR expression as a consequence of impaired histone acetylation and through recruitment of the corepressor.[68] Although its mechanism remains unclear, it has been hypothesized that the 19 KDa lipoprotein induced TLR2 signaling, which can be responsible for the expression/activation/repression of these identified transcription factors.[69,70] The precise mechanisms involved require further investigation. One more protein, that is, early secreted antigen (ESAT-6), is known to play an important role in the reduction of IFN-γ-induced histone H3K4 methylation and histone acetylation at the CIITA pI locus in *M.tb*-infected macrophages. Inhibition of type I and type IV CIITA expression by ESAT6 is by both TLR2-dependent and independent pathways.[71] This study further confirms that methylation and acetylation plays an important role in *M.tb* infection and its survival.[71] Apart from ESAT6, one more *M.tb* protein plays an important role in epigenetic modification to promote its own survival. *M.tb* secreted enhanced intracellular survival (Eis) protein, known to acetylate the histone proteins in macrophages infected with *Mycobacterium smegmatis,* which increases its survival.[72] Additional mechanisms must be determined to exactly understand how *M.tb* induces the repressor recruitment to this

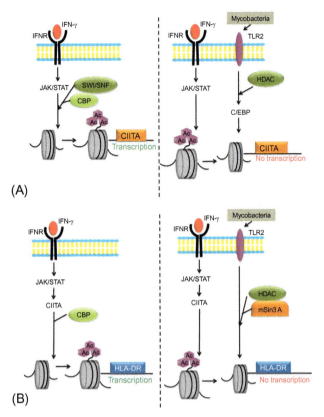

Fig. 4.5 *M. tuberculosis* inhibits (A) IFNγ induced genes like CIITA and (B) HLA-DR through histone modification and chromatin remodeling at specific promoter.

promoter in a highly specific way. Different strains of *M.tb* follow different mechanisms of gene regulation. For example, optimal immune activation by a drug-sensitive *M.tb* strain (CDC1551) is sufficient to clear the pathogens from the host, however, drug-resistant *M.tb* strain (HN878) can suboptimally induce immune activation to induce overexpression of genes involved in host lipid metabolism, hence, enabling improved intracellular survival of HN878 bacilli.[73] Precise molecular details about these differences are still unclear. This necessitates further study to decipher the epigenetic changes happening in the host and *M.tb* that makes one strain drug-sensitive and others resistant.

Experimental studies have shown that, via epigenetic reprogramming of monocytes, BCG induces nonspecific protection from reinfection.

Protection of severe combined immunodeficiency SCID mice from disseminated candidiasis has been noticed in BCG-vaccinated mice through induction of NOD2-mediated histone methylation (H3K4me3) in mononuclear phagocytes.[74] Chandran et al. showed the role of HDAC1 and acetylation of H3 in survival of *M.tb* inside a host. *M.tb* infection significantly induces HADC1-mediated suppression of IL12B gene expression and downregulates H3 acetylation in infected macrophages.[75] Hypoacetylation of H3 suppresses the expression of Th1 cells by suppressing regulating gene expression, hence increasing the survival of *M.tb* inside the host.

A group of researchers showed that overexpression of matrix metalloproteinases (MMP), a host enzyme critical for the development of cavitation, during TB is also caused because of epigenetic mechanisms involving histone acetylation. It has been proven that HDAC and HAT activity is necessary for inducible expression of MMP-1 and MMP-3 in *M.tb*-infected macrophages.[76] In recent years, it has been found that *M.tb* infection and susceptibility is also related to methylation of the vitamin D receptor gene.[77]

Each of these studies show the correlation between *M.*tb susceptibility inside a host and the level of methylation status of the host. Further understanding is required for deducing the epigenetic reprogramming of immunity during *M.tb* infection, which could be potentially used for designing novel and effective vaccines and adjuvants.

ROLE OF RNA INTERFERENCE IN TB INFECTION

miRNAs play a central role in many developmental processes like differentiation, apoptosis, and oncogenesis. Apart from normal developmental processes, their role has also been studied in many diseases. Focusing on TB, multiple studies have shown the dynamics of miRNA expression in TB patients. Fu et al. have shown differential expression of 92 miRNA (59 upregulated miRNA and 33 downregulated miRNA) in TB patients compared with the uninfected individuals.[78] These data suggest that miRNA can be targeted as a novel biomarker for the diagnosis of active TB.[78] A recent study has shown the role of miR115 in *M.tb* infection. miR115 expression is upregulated in *Mycobacterium bovis*-infected macrophages, and it diversifies macrophage signaling, which is essential for pathogenesis and survival of *M.tb*.[79]

MicroRNA analysis of human monocyte-derived macrophages infected with several *Mycobacterium avium hominissuis* strains by means of microarrays as well as quantitative reverse transcription PCR (qRT-PCR) have shown the role of miRNA 155, miRNA 146a, and miRNA 886-5p during infection.[80]

Interferon-γ (IFN-γ) role in immune response against intracellular pathogens is well known. Recently, it has been observed that miRNA 29 suppresses IFN-γ production by directly targeting IFN-γ mRNA in natural killer cells, CD4[+] T cells, and CD8[+] T cells. Hence, miRNA29 is responsible for suppression of the immune system during *M.tb* infection.[81]

M.tb-infected human dendritic cells (DCs) also showed changes in their miRNA profile. Genome-wide expression profiling showed that approximately 40% of miRNAs were differently expressed in *M.tb*-infected DCs. It has been found that 155 miRNAs were differentially expressed upon infection, of which 64 were upregulated and 91 were downregulated. The most differentially expressed miRNAs upon infection include, among others, the upregulated miR-155, miR-132, and miR-29a, and the downregulated miR-361-5p, miR-185, and miR-27a. These miRNAs are involved in the modulation of immune functions.[82]

All these results highlight the critical role of miRNAs in *M.tb*-infected cells and lay the foundation of a new field in epigenetic research focused on the role of miRNA in pathophysiology of TB. Additional mechanisms are likely yet to be discovered regarding the relationship between miRNAs in TB immunity, infection, disease, and latency.

ROLE OF DNA METHYLATION IN TB INFECTION AND ITS SURVIVAL INSIDE A HOST

The role of DNA methylation has been extensively studied with respect to TB infection. Barreiro LB et al. showed marked difference in methylation profile of DCs before and after *M.tb* infection using single base pair resolution data.[83] These methylation were observed at CpG shores and distal regulatory regions or enhancers rather than in CpG islands and gene promoters.[83] Similar findings were made with infected macrophages where the results were the same.[84] One such data is provided by Ip et al., where they showed a marked difference in the methylation at the promoter region of the IL 17 receptor gene in *M.tb*-infected human macrophages.[84] Recently, studies revealed that infection with Beijing/W *M.tb* strains causes IL6R, IL4R, and IL17R gene hypermethylation in infected macrophages.[85] In 2006, Wei et al. also showed that *M.tb* infection activates the NLRP3 inflammosome in macrophages and dendritic cells through DNA methylation modification.[86] It was shown that *M.tb* infection demethylates the promoter region of NLRP3 inflammamosome, which increases the secretion of inflammatory cytokines.[86] This epigenetic tag favors the host immune system to eradicate the pathogen from the body. These studies provide strong evidence that DNA methylation plays an important role in TB susceptibility.

FUTURE PROSPECTS

M.tb is a highly tenacious organism that is evolving at a faster pace than its human host. *M.tb* can escape host immune responses via multiple pathways such as inhibition of phagosome maturation, inhibition of inflammatory cytokine production, etc. Recent research has added epigenetic modifications as another immune evasion mechanism employed by *M.tb* to promote its survival inside the host. Unraveling these epigenetic tags likely will be important in the development of efficient vaccines and new therapeutic drugs against TB.

REFERENCES

1. Goldberg AD, Allis CD, Bernstein E. Epigenetics: a landscape takes shape. *Cell.* 2007;128(4):635–638.
2. Bird A. Perceptions of epigenetics. *Nature.* 2007;447(7143):396–398.
3. Weinhold B. Epigenetics: the science of change. *Environ Health Perspect.* 2006;114(3): 160–167.
4. Cairns BR. The logic of chromatin architecture and remodelling at promoters. *Nature.* 2009;461(7261):193–198.
5. Jenuwein T, Allis CD. Translating the histone code. *Science.* 2001;293(5532):1074–1080.
6. Kouzarides T. Chromatin modifications and their function. *Cell.* 2007;128(4):693–705.
7. Mehler MF. Epigenetic principles and mechanisms underlying nervous system functions in health and disease. *Prog Neurobiol.* 2008;86(4):305–341.
8. Bhavsar AP, Guttman JA, Finlay BB. Manipulation of host-cell pathways by bacterial pathogens. *Nature.* 2007;449(7164):827–834.
9. Webster JP. Natural history of host-parasite interactions. In: *Advances in Parasitology.* vol. 68. Dunfermline: Academic Press/Better World Books Ltd; 2009.
10. Hamon MA, Cossart P. Histone modifications and chromatin remodeling during bacterial infections. *Cell Host Microbe.* 2008;4(2):100–109.
11. Lefevre T, Lebarbenchon C, Gauthier-Clerc M, Misse D, Poulin R, Thomas F. The ecological significance of manipulative parasites. *Trends Ecol Evol.* 2009;24(1):41–48.
12. Paschos K, Allday MJ. Epigenetic reprogramming of host genes in viral and microbial pathogenesis. *Trends Microbiol.* 2010;18(10):439–447.
13. Ribet D, Cossart P. Post-translational modifications in host cells during bacterial infection. *FEBS Lett.* 2010;584(13):2748–2758.
14. Kay S, Hahn S, Marois E, Hause G, Bonas U. A bacterial effector acts as a plant transcription factor and induces a cell size regulator. *Science.* 2007;318(5850):648–651.
15. WHO. *Global tuberculosis report.* Geneva: WHO Press; 2016.
16. Cole E, Cook C. Characterization of infectious aerosols in health care facilities: an aid to effective engineering controls and preventive strategies. *Am J Infect Control.* 1998;26(4):453–464.

17. Espinal MA, Laszlo A, Simonsen L, et al. Global trends in resistance to antituberculosis drugs: World Health Organization-International Union against Tuberculosis and Lung Disease Working Group on Anti-Tuberculosis Drug Resistance Surveillance. *N Engl J Med.* 2001;344(17):1294–1303.

18. Pablos-Méndez A, Raviglione MC, Laszlo A, et al. Global surveillance for antituberculosis-drug resistance, 1994–1997: World Health Organization-International Union against Tuberculosis and Lung Disease Working Group on Anti-Tuberculosis Drug Resistance Surveillance. *N Engl J Med.* 1998;338(23):1641–1649.

19. World Health Organization. *Anti-tuberculosis drug resistance in the world.* The WHO/IUATLD global project on anti-tuberculosis drug resistance surveillance report no. 3, Geneva: World Health Organization; 2004.16–20.

20. Almeida Da Silva PE, Palomino JC. Molecular basis and mechanisms of drug resistance in Mycobacterium tuberculosis: classical and new drugs. *J Antimicrob Chemother.* 2011;66(7):1417–1430.

21. Davies J. Origins and evolution of antibiotic resistance. *Microbiologia.* 1996;74(3):9–16.

22. Gillespie SH. Evolution of drug resistance in Mycobacterium tuberculosis: clinical and molecular perspective. *Antimicrob Agents Chemother.* 2002;46(2):267–274.

23. Shah NS, Wright A, Bai GH, et al. Worldwide emergence of extensively drug-resistant tuberculosis. *Emerg Infect Dis.* 2007;13(3):380–387.

24. Velayati AA, Farnia P, Masjedi MR, et al. Totally drug-resistant tuberculosis strains: evidence of adaptation at the cellular level. *Eur Respir J.* 2009;34(5):1202–1203.

25. Flynn JL, Chan J. Immunology of tuberculosis. *Annu Rev Immunol.* 2001;19:93–129.

26. Koul A, Arnoult E, Lounis N, Guillemont J, Andries K. The challenge of new drug discovery for tuberculosis. *Nature.* 2011;469(7331):483–490.

27. McGhee JD, Ginder GD. Specific DNA methylation sites in the vicinity of the chicken beta-globin genes. *Nature.* 1979;280(5721):419–420.

28. Bhutani N, Burns DM, Blau HM. DNA demethylation dynamics. *Cell.* 2011;146(6):866–872.

29. Bird A. The essentials of DNA methylation. *Cell.* 1992;70(1):5–8.

30. Fatemi M, Hermann A, Gowher H, Jeltsch A. Dnmt3a and Dnmt1 functionally cooperate during de novo methylation of DNA. *Eur J Biochem.* 2002;269(20):4981–4984.

31. Deaton AM, Bird A. CpG islands and the regulation of transcription. *Genes Dev.* 2011;25(10):1010–1022.

32. Siedlecki P, Zielenkiewicz P. Mammalian DNA methyltransferases. *Acta Biochim Pol.* 2006;53(2):245–256.

33. Woodcock CL, Dimitrov S. Higher-order structure of chromatin and chromosomes. *Curr Opin Genet Dev.* 2001;11(2):130–135.

34. Alberts BJA, Lewis J, Raff M, Roberts K, Walter P. Chromosomal DNA and its packaging in the chromatin fiber. In: *Molecular Biology of the Cell.* 4th ed. New York: Garland Science; 2002.

35. Kornberg RD, Lorch Y. Twenty-five years of the nucleosome, fundamental particle of the eukaryote chromosome. *Cell.* 1999;98(3):285–294.

36. Carl W. Chromatin remodeling and the control of gene expression. *J Biol Chem.* 1997;272(45):281.

37. Cosgrove MS, Boeke JD, Wolberger C. Regulated nucleosome mobility and the histone code. *Nat Struct Mol Biol.* 2004;11(11):1037–1043.

38. Goll MG, Bestor TH. Histone modification and replacement in chromatin activation. *Genes Dev.* 2002;16(14):1739–1742.

39. Grant PA. A tale of histone modifications. *Genome Biol.* 2001;2(4):REVIEWS0003.

40. Shahbazian MD, Grunstein M. Functions of site-specific histone acetylation and deacetylation. *Annu Rev Biochem.* 2007;76:75–100.

41. The ENCODE Project Consortium. Identification and analysis of functional elements in 1% of the human genome by the ENCODE pilot project. *Nature.* 2007;447(7146):799–816.
42. Krivtsov AV, Feng Z, Lemieux ME, et al. H3K79 methylation profiles define murine and human MLL-AF4 leukemias. *Cancer Cell.* 2008;14(5):355–368.
43. Groth A, Rocha W, Verreault A, Almouzni G. Chromatin challenges during DNA replication and repair. *Cell.* 2007;128(4):721–733.
44. Peterson CL, Laniel MA. Histones and histone modifications. *Curr Biol.* 2004;14(14): 546–551.
45. Bannister AJ, Zegerman P, Partridge JF, et al. Selective recognition of methylated lysine 9 on histone H3 by the HP1 chromo domain. *Nature.* 2001;410(6824):120–124.
46. Wysocka J, Swigut T, Xiao H, et al. A PHD finger of NURF couples histone H3 lysine 4 trimethylation with chromatin remodelling. *Nature.* 2006;442(7098):86–90.
47. Zhou Y, Kim J, Yuan X, Braun T. Epigenetic modifications of stem cells: a paradigm for the control of cardiac progenitor cells. *Circ Res.* 2011;109(9):1067–1081.
48. Chen ZX, Riggs AD. DNA methylation and demethylation in mammals. *J Biol Chem.* 2011;286(21):18347–18353.
49. Feinberg AP, Tycko B. The history of cancer epigenetics. *Nat Rev Cancer.* 2004;4(2): 143–153.
50. Ruttenburg A, Li H, Patel DJ, Allis CD. Multivalent engagement of chromatin modifications by linked binding modules. *Nat Rev Mol Cell Biol.* 2007;8(12):983–994.
51. Bentwich I, Avniel A, Karov Y, et al. Identification of hundreds of conserved and nonconserved human microRNAs. *Nat Genet.* 2005;37(7):766–770.
52. Lewis BP, Burge CB, Bartel DP. Conserved seed pairing, often flanked by adenosines, indicates that thousands of human genes are microRNA targets. *Cell.* 2005;120(1):15–20.
53. Sontheimer EJ, Carthew RW. Silence from within: endogenous siRNAs and miRNAs. *Cell.* 2005;122(1):9–12.
54. Ambros V. The functions of animal microRNAs. *Nature.* 2004;431(7006):350–355.
55. Calin GA, Sevignani C, Dumitru CD, et al. Human microRNA genes are frequently located at fragile sites and genomic regions involved in cancers. *Proc Natl Acad Sci USA.* 2004;101(9):2999–3004.
56. Borchert GM, Lanier W, Davidson BL. RNA polymerase III transcribes human microRNAs. *Nat Struct Mol Biol.* 2006;13(12):1097–1101.
57. Cai X, Hagedorn CH, Cullen BR. Human microRNAs are processed from capped, polyadenylated transcripts that can also function as mRNAs. *RNA.* 2004;10(12): 1957–1966.
58. Lee Y, Jeon K, Lee JT, Kim S. Kim VN. MicroRNA maturation: stepwise processing and subcellular localization. *EMBO J.* 2002;21:4663–4670.
59. Lee Y, Kim M, Han J, et al. MicroRNA genes are transcribed by RNA polymerase II. *EMBO J.* 2004;23(20):4051–4060.
60. Bartel DP. MicroRNAs: genomics, biogenesis, mechanism, and function. *Cell.* 2004;116(2):281–297.
61. Cheng AM, Byrom MW, Shelton J, Ford LP. Antisense inhibition of human miRNAs and indications for an involvement of miRNA in cell growth and apoptosis. *Nucleic Acids Res.* 2005;33(4):1290–1297.
62. Hua Z, Lv Q, Ye W, et al. MiRNA-directed regulation of VEGF and other angiogenic factors under hypoxia. *PLoS One.* 2006;1:e116.
63. Boehm U, Klamp T, Groot M, Howard JC. Cellular responses to interferon-gamma. *Annu Rev Immunol.* 1997;15:749–795.
64. Kincaid EZ, Ernst JD. Mycobacterium tuberculosis exerts gene-selective inhibition of transcriptional responses to IFN-gamma without inhibiting STAT1 function. *J Immunol.* 2003;171(4):2042–2049.

65. Kretsovali A, Agalioti T, Spilianakis C, Tzortzakaki E, Merika M, Papamatheakis J. Involvement of CREB binding protein in expression of major histocompatibility complex class II genes via interaction with the class II transactivator. *Mol Cell Biol.* 1998;18(11):6777–6783.

66. Pattenden SG, Klose R, Karaskov E, Bremner R. Interferon-gamma-induced chromatin remodeling at the CIITA locus is BRG1 dependent. *EMBO J.* 2002;21(8):1978–1986.

67. Hamon AM, Cossart P. Histone modification and chromatin remodeling during bacterial infections. *Cell Host Microbe.* 2008;4(2):100–109.

68. Wang Y, Curry HM, Zwilling BS, Lafuse WP. Mycobacteria inhibition of IFN-gamma induced HLA-DR gene expression by up-regulating histone deacetylation at the promoter region in human THP-1 monocytic cells. *J Immunol.* 2005;174(9):5687–5694.

69. Pennini ME, Liu Y, Yang J, Croniger CM, Boom WH, Harding CV. CCAAT/ enhancer-binding protein beta and delta binding to CIITA promoters is associated with the inhibition of CIITA expression in response to Mycobacterium tuberculosis 19-kDa lipoprotein. *J Immunol.* 2007;179(10):6910–6918.

70. Pennini ME, Pai RK, Schultz DC, Boom WH, Harding CV. Mycobacterium tuberculosis 19-kDa lipoprotein inhibits IFN-gamma-induced chromatin remodeling of MHC-2TA by TLR2 and MAPK signaling. *J Immunol.* 2006;176(7):4323–4330.

71. Kumar P, Agarwal R, Siddiqui I, Vora H, Das G, Sharma P. ESAT6 differentially inhibits IFN-gamma-inducible class II transactivator isoforms in both a TLR2-dependent and -independent manner. *Immunol Cell Biol.* 2012;90(4):411–420.

72. Crossman DK. *Characterization of a Novel Acetyltransferase Found Only in Pathogenic Strains of Mycobacterium Tuberculosis.* Tuscaloosa, AL: University of Alabama; 2007. PhD Thesis.

73. Koo MS, Subbian S, Kaplan G. Strain specific transcriptional response in Mycobacterium tuberculosis infected macrophages. *Cell Commun Signal.* 2012;10(1):2.

74. Kleinnijenhuis J, Quintin J, Preijers F, et al. Bacille Calmette-Guerin induces NOD2-dependent nonspecific protection from reinfection via epigenetic reprogramming of monocytes. *Proc Natl Acad Sci USA.* 2012;109(43):17537–17542.

75. Chandran A, Antony CL, Mundayoor S, Natarajan K, Kumar AR. Mycobacterium tuberculosis infection induces HDAC1-mediated suppression of IL-12B gene expression in macrophages. *Front Cell Infect Microbiol.* 2015;5:90.

76. Moores RC, Brilha S, Schutgens F, Elkington PT, Friedland JS. Epigenetic regulation of matrix metalloproteinase 1 and 3 expression in Mycobacterium tuberculosis infection. *Front Immunol.* 2017;8:602.

77. Andraos C, Koorsen G, Knight JC, Bornman L. Vitamin D receptor gene methylation is associated with ethnicity, tuberculosis, and TaqI polymorphism. *Hum Immunol.* 2011;72(3):262–268.

78. Fu Y, Yi Z, Wu X, Li J, Xu F. Circulating microRNAs in patients with active pulmonary tuberculosis. *J Clin Microbiol.* 2011;49(12):4246–4251.

79. Ghorpade DS, Leyland R, Kurowska-Stolarska M, Patil SA, Balaji KN. MicroRNA-155 is required for Mycobacterium bovis BCG-mediated apoptosis of macrophages. *Mol Cell Biol.* 2012;32(12):2239–2253.

80. Sharbati J, Lewin A, Kutz-Lohroff B, Kamal E, Einspanier R, Sharbati S. Integrated microRNA-mRNA-analysis of human monocyte derived macrophages upon Mycobacterium avium subsp. hominissuis infection. *PLoS One.* 2011;6(5):e20258.

81. Ma F, Xu S, Liu X, et al. The microRNA miR-29 controls innate and adaptive immune responses to intracellular bacterial infection by targeting interferon-gamma. *Nat Immunol.* 2011;12(9):861–869.

82. Siddle KJ, Deschamps M, Tailleux L, et al. A genomic portrait of the genetic architecture and regulatory impact of microRNA expression in response to infection. *Genome Res.* 2014;24(5):850–859.

83. Barreiro LB, Tailleaux APL, Yotova V, et al. *Widespread changes in DNA methylation at CpG island shores and distal regulatory regions in response to a bacterial infection*; 2013, http://www.ashg.org/2013meeting/abstracts/fulltext/f130123390.htm.
84. Zheng L, Leung ET, Wong HK, et al. Unraveling methylation changes of host macrophages in Mycobacterium tuberculosis infection. *Tuberculosis*. 2016;98:139–148.
85. Zheng L, Leung E, Lee N, et al. Differential microRNA expression in human macrophages with Mycobacterium tuberculosis infection of Beijing/W and nonBeijing/W strain types. *PLoS One*. 2015;10(6):e0126018.
86. Wei M, Wang L, Wu T, et al. NLRP3 activation was regulated by DNA methylation modification during Mycobacterium tuberculosis infection. *Biomed Res Int*. 2016, https://doi.org/10.1155/2016/4323281.

FURTHER READING

Berger SL, Kouzarides T, Shiekhattar R, Shilatifard A. An operational definition of epigenetics. *Genes Dev*. 2009;23(7):781–783.

CHAPTER 5

Mycobacterium Bovis Bacille Calmette-Guerin Vaccination: Can Biomarkers Predict Efficacy?

Hazel M. Dockrell

Department of Immunology and Infection, London School of Hygiene & Tropical Medicine, London, United Kingdom

Contents

INTRODUCTION

The BCG vaccine provides protection against the disseminated forms of TB in children, such as TB meningitis.[1,2] It is also a cheap and cost-effective vaccine.[3] However, it only provides variable protection against pulmonary TB in adults.[2,4] The search is therefore on for a more effective vaccine against TB, particularly to protect against the pulmonary infections that spread the disease. In 2017, the TB vaccine pipeline contained 19 candidates that were in preclinical studies or in phase I, phase IIa, or phase IIb trials (see http://www.aeras.org/pages/global-portfolio). Some of these vaccine candidates aim to replace BCG, for example, with a safe *Mycobacterium tuberculosis* mutant called MTBVAC,[5] whereas others are recombinant BCG vaccines that are hoped to be more protective than the current BCG vaccine strains.[6,7] The majority of the vaccine candidates are designed to be given as a boosting vaccination following BCG, either delivered by a viral vector or as proteins in adjuvant. If protective biosignatures induced following BCG vaccination could be identified, this might accelerate the development of a protective TB vaccine.[8,9]

The Value of BCG and TNF in Autoimmunity
https://doi.org/10.1016/B978-0-12-814603-3.00005-7

What BCG does in terms of the immune responses it induces is also of great interest in terms of the potential use of the BCG vaccine as an immune modulator in autoimmune diseases. This chapter will therefore discuss progress toward identifying protective biosignatures, the specific and nonspecific cytokine responses BCG vaccination induces, and what has been learned about why it induces such variable protection against pulmonary TB. In all these cases, the knowledge learned has the potential to accelerate the development of a better vaccine for TB, as well as provide insights into BCG's potential role as an immunotherapy for autoimmune diseases.

BIOMARKERS THAT PREDICT PROTECTION

BCG vaccination induces scar formation and a Th1 cell response in infants.[10] Measurement of interferon-γ (IFNγ)—the signature Th1 cytokine secreted in response to BCG itself or to crossreactive mycobacterial antigen preparations such as *Mycobacterium tuberculosis* purified protein derivative (PPD)—can be used as a robust readout of immunogenicity in UK adolescents and infants.[11,12] However, although mice that cannot make or respond to IFNγ are more susceptible to *M. tuberculosis* infection and are unable to control the growth of the mycobacteria,[13] directly measuring IFNγ is not a readout of protection in mouse models.[14,15] In fact, quantitation of IFNγ secretion in response to peptides from *M. tuberculosis* antigens is the basis of two commercial assays for detection of *M. tuberculosis* infection or TB disease: QuantiFERON-TB Gold In Tube (or the newer QuantiFERON-TB Plus) and T.SPOT-TB. Thus, it is generally assumed that, although adding IFNγ to murine macrophages increases their ability to control mycobacterial growth, IFNγ is necessary but not by itself sufficient for protection.

It was hoped that polyfunctional T cells that produce IFNγ, TNFα, and IL-2 might be a better correlate of protection.[16] In addition to the potentially synergistic effects of having IL-2 and TNFα production, as well as that of IFNγ, a study by Darrah et al.[17] showed that such polyfunctional T cells produced more IFNγ per cell than those T cells producing IFNγ alone. Mycobacteria-specific polyfunctional T cells are induced when immunologically naive infants in the United Kingdom are given BCG at about 3 to 4 months of age, measuring the responses induced in response to PPD 4 or 12 months postvaccination.[18,19] Age-matched unvaccinated infants, a valuable control group that is not available except in countries where some but not all babies receive BCG vaccination, show few if any of these mycobacterial antigen-specific polyfunctional T cells. These studies in low TB incidence settings cannot, however, have development of or protection from disease as an endpoint. Thus, in recent years, a series of studies have been performed in South Africa, a setting that has an extremely high incidence of TB, which makes it an ideal setting for vaccine trials.[20] A large study performed in Worcester close to Cape Town, which provided a baseline for new prime boost vaccination studies, recruited enough infants (a total of 5726) to have detection of TB disease as an endpoint, enabling immune responses in those who progressed to TB disease within 2 years to be compared with either household or community controls. This landmark study used rigorous diagnostic criteria with investigations that included gastric lavage to confirm TB in the children, which is normally a diagnostic challenge.[21] However, there was no difference in the frequencies of polyfunctional T cells, in this case measured in whole blood, in response to stimulation with BCG itself at 10 weeks postvaccination, with subsequent development of TB,[22] nor were there differences in the frequencies of T cells making IFNγ alone, or T cells making IFNγ with just TNFα, or IFNγ with just IL-2. It is worth noting, however, that the frequency of all the cell types studied were very variable in all three groups. A marked heterogeneity in cytokine responses was also observed in BCG-vaccinated Gambian infants with IFNγ, IL-5, and IL-13 secretion induced by stimulation of diluted whole blood with PPD, BCG Ag85, a short term culture filtrate of *M. tuberculosis*, or killed *M. tuberculosis* measured by ELISA.[23] A recent review considered the evidence that mycobacteria-specific polyfunctional T cells are associated with protection against TB.[16] Mycobacteria-specific polyfunctional T cells can be induced by vaccine candidates of different types including live mycobacterial vaccines, viral-vector delivered vaccines, and recombinant protein vaccines in adjuvant. However, although there are some studies that show an association of polyfunctional T cells induced by vaccination with vaccine efficacy in the mouse model, there are other murine studies as well as the study by Kagina et al. in South African infants[22] that fail to show such an association.[16]

A subsequent study on the same cohort of South African infants used a biology systems approach.[24] No specific, cellular, or cytokine signatures of TB risk were present in supernatants from the whole blood cultures stimulated with BCG, measured in a multiplex bead array assay, nor were differences in expression of cytotoxic T cell markers, T cell proliferation, or frequencies of myeloid or lymphoid cells detected. Perhaps more surprisingly, there was no gene expression signature that discriminated between the infants who subsequently progressed to disease when compared with the household controls, comparing signatures in peripheral blood mononuclear cells (PBMC) stimulated with BCG for 12 h in infants at 10 weeks of age, having subtracted the gene expression in unstimulated cultures. What this analysis did show was that both cases and controls could be divided into two subgroups or clusters based on their BCG-stimulated gene expression, having subtracted gene expression in unstimulated cultures, although subsequent analysis showed that unstimulated PBMC cultures also divided into the same clusters. Genes characteristic of myeloid cells and antiinflammatory gene sets were found associated with one cluster, and genes associated with T cells were upregulated in the second cluster. Further analysis indicated that infants with either the highest or the lowest rations of monocytes to T cells were at greater risk of developing TB. This degree of complexity and heterogeneity may help explain why in such studies it has been hard to identify correlates of protection and why, for example, the earlier study by Kagina et al.[22] had showed such heterogeneity in the frequencies of polyfunctional T cells.

The only other published study that has been of sufficient size to have progression to TB in BCG-vaccinated infants as an outcome used infants from the MVA85A phase 2b efficacy trial.[25] The MVA85A vaccine given as a boosting vaccine at 4 to 6 months of age failed to induce significant protective efficacy when compared with the placebo group that received Candin, although the MVA85A vaccine was able induce IFNγ-secreting cells to the Ag85A peptides.[26] When responses in 53 infants who developed TB were compared with those in 205 matched controls, all of whom received BCG only, activated T cells that expressed HLA-DR were higher in infants who progressed to disease and also in TB progressers from another adolescent cohort.[25] Within the group of infants who subsequently progressed to disease, the rate of progression was faster in those who had the highest numbers of HLA-DR expressing (activated) T cells, whereas the rate of progression was slower in those with the highest numbers of BCG-stimulated IFNγ spot-forming cells detected in an ELISPOT assay.

Further studies are needed to clarify why IFNγ-producing cells were associated with protection in the study by Fletcher et al.[25] but not in that of Kagina et al.[22] Although both studies were performed in BCG-vaccinated South African infants, there were differences in the methodology and the age at which they were studied. In the study by Fletcher et al.,[25] the infants were older when bled, 4 to 6 months of age rather than 10 weeks of age as in the study by Kagina et al.[22] The Fletcher study had a larger sample size and used three controls matched to each infant.[25] Thus, at present, although it is clear that protection requires IFNγ-producing T cells, confirmation is needed as to whether they provide a correlate of protection.

BACK TO BASICS AND GROWTH INHIBITION OF BCG

Against the background of the complexities and heterogeneities that these human studies reveal, and without a confirmed correlate of protection, there has been a recent move back to the use of functional assays that do not presuppose which immune mechanisms are involved in protection. One example of such an assay that has received considerable attention is the mycobacterial growth inhibition assay (MGIA).[27–30] It seems a given that, if BCG vaccination is able to induce significant protection against TB, it should increase the ability to inhibit the growth of, if not kill, BCG and *M. tuberculosis* itself.

The earlier forms of these assays were performed using PBMC, often using monocytes and lymphocytes that were matured or activated separately before the putative effector T cells were added to infected monocyte-derived macrophages.[31] Quantitation of the mycobacteria was usually performed by counting colony-forming units. As larger blood volumes were required, these assays were research tools and not fit for use in large vaccine trials where only small blood samples and thus limited numbers of peripheral blood mononuclear cells would be available. In these assays, growth inhibition was not always associated with production of IFNγ,[32,33] although BCG vaccination usually induced significant antimycobacterial activity.[32] To make assessment of mycobacterial growth inhibition simpler, an assay that used recombinant BCG expressing the *lux* gene was developed.[34] Another simple assay exploits the Bactec MGIT machine.[27] In this case, whole blood samples or PBMC are cultured with a fixed inoculum of BCG or *M. tuberculosis* for 4 days before the remaining mycobacteria are recovered from cultures and added to a Bactec tube. Comparison of the time to positivity of these test tubes is compared with that of a mycobacteria control tube in which the original inoculum of mycobacteria is added straight to a Bactec tube without incubation. This assay can demonstrate marked growth inhibition of mycobacteria in UK BCG-vaccinated infants 4 months after vaccination compared with unvaccinated infants.[18] Interestingly, some infants lose their ability to inhibit the growth of BCG by 12 months postvaccination whereas others retain it. Although as previously noted, polyfunctional T cells have not proved to be a readout of BCG-induced protection in South African infants, in this much smaller study in the United Kingdom, there was an association between polyfunctional T cells and growth inhibition of BCG.[18] In this assay, the addition of the immunosuppressive cytokines IL-10 or TGFβ inhibits mycobacterial growth inhibition, yet their inhibition using blocking antibodies enhances it (Anwar, Dockrell, unpublished results). Multicenter studies have improved the MGIA protocol and made it more reproducible, but there is still an interesting variability in growth inhibition shown by different individuals, whether infants or adults. Again, some of this may reflect the variability in numbers of monocytes or in the monocyte:lymphocyte ratios in these individuals.[24]

WHAT INFLUENCES THE BIOMARKERS INDUCED BY BCG VACCINATION IN DIFFERENT SETTINGS?

Vaccines do not always induce equivalent immunity in different geographic locations.[35] There are precedents where vaccines designed to protect against pathogens in the gut have shown variable protection in African or Asian countries compared with the United States, for example, the Rotavirus vaccine.[36] These geographic variations may reflect the burden of intestinal infections experienced by children in Africa or Asia, or other environmental or maternal factors. The BCG vaccine also induces variable protection, with the best protection observed in countries of greater latitude and less efficacy in countries nearer the equator.[2,4,37] Studies comparing BCG-vaccinated adolescents in the United Kingdom with adolescents and young adults in Malawi showed that the baseline IFNγ responses to PPD of *M. tuberculosis* were markedly different in these two settings, with most Malawians already presensitized to mycobacterial antigens,[11] even though the majority did not make an IFNγ response to the more specific *M. tuberculosis* ESAT6 antigen in a 7-day diluted whole blood assay.[38] One year following vaccination, there was a marked increase in IFNγ responses to PPD in those vaccinated in the United Kingdom, whereas responses in the vaccinated Malawians were not significantly different from those in the unvaccinated controls receiving placebo.[11]

More surprisingly, the responses in BCG-vaccinated infants in the two settings were also different.[12] In the United Kingdom, unvaccinated infants could be studied, as not all UK infants are offered BCG vaccination. These unvaccinated UK infants were largely unresponsive to PPD even at 1 year of age, whereas BCG-vaccinated infants in the United Kingdom made a strong IFNγ response at 3 months postvaccination that only reduced slightly by 1 year postvaccination. Age-matched BCG-vaccinated infants in Malawi, given the same BCG vaccine, did not make as strong an IFNγ response as the equivalent UK BCG-vaccinated infants.

One common explanation for such variability in responses is that it results from exposure to environmental or nontuberculous mycobacteria (NTMs). A panel of PPDs from these environmental mycobacteria were used to test induction of IFNγ responses in a 7-day diluted whole blood assay in the adolescent and young adult studies and confirmed that cross-reactive responses to PPDs from NTMs were present in Malawi, with a trend toward improved vaccine-induced responses in those with lower NTM responses.[39] The extensive cross-reactivity of the antigens shared between most mycobacteria makes it very challenging to identify which environmental mycobacteria individuals are exposed to with relatively few "specific" NTM antigens identified to date,[40] but comparing responses to PPDs from different NTMs may be useful.[39] Different NTMs may have different effects, with live replicating NTMs having the greatest effect on the BCG response[41]; however immunologically naïve infants will not have been exposed to environmental mycobacteria if vaccinated soon after birth at a time when they are not exposed to soil and are exclusively breast fed. Exposure to NTMs postvaccination may be important as well as exposure prevaccination.[42] Restricting BCG vaccination to those lacking a PPD response detected by skin testing improves BCG-induced protection.[2]

The studies in Malawian infants revealed another variation in responses associated with seasonality. Infants born in the hot/dry season gave stronger IFNγ responses than those born in the wet/rainy season.[12] A weaker association of IFNγ responses associated with seasonality was observed in the United Kingdom. Such variation has been observed for responses to other vaccines given slightly later in infancy or to young children; in northern countries where nutrition is not suboptimal, this may reflect intercurrent infections. In a country such as Malawi, food may be limiting at certain times of year due to poor harvests, limited availability, or price rises. However, such variation may have its roots not just at the time when immune responses are measured or when the vaccine was administered, but during conception or in utero. Seasonal effects on immune responses, as well as variation in gene expression and in blood composition, have been observed in infants studied in the Gambia.[43–45] Another seasonal factor that could impact on the BCG-induced immune responses measured in these assays may be the prevalence of infections, such as with malaria.[46]

Another source of variability in responses to BCG vaccination may be the epigenetic marks present on the DNA of different individuals, some of which may be determined in utero by factors such as maternal nutrition.[47] The extent of gene transcription varies with DNA methylation and histone modification, with patterns of response passed on not only to daughter cells but from mother to offspring. Thus the magnitude of an IFNγ response following BCG vaccination may vary not only with the number of mycobacteria-specific T cells an individual has, and whether they have the MHC alleles required to present key peptides to these T cells, but also on how a series of genes has been modified epigenetically. When DNA methylation is compared in high and low IFNγ responder infants following BCG vaccination, the patterns of DNA methylation are different in the two groups, and pathway analysis reveals that, as well as genes associated with immune signaling, other genes involved in cellular processes such as membrane ion flux are also differentially methylated and may influence the response to BCG (Hasso-Agopsowicz, Scriba, Hanekom, Dockrell, and Smith, manuscript submitted for publication). BCG vaccination also induces alterations in innate immunity, with altered cytokine production in response to nonspecific innate stimuli.[48,49] This phenomenon has been termed innate memory or trained immunity and relies upon the epigenetic modification of histones to program monocytes for enhanced responses.[50] Epigenetic changes have also been found that associate with control of mycobacterial replication.[51] This new approach may help identify further underlying differences in high and low cytokine responders following BCG vaccination.

Another possible maternal influence on the immune response in a BCG-vaccinated infant may result from the mother's own mycobacterial exposure. In TB-endemic countries, many adults have a latent TB infection (LTBI), and it is possible that mothers with LTBI might give birth to infants already presensitized to mycobacterial antigens, although one study in South Africa had not documented a marked effect of mycobacterial exposure of the mother.[52] A recent study in Uganda compared immune responses in BCG-vaccinated infants born to mothers with or without LTBI.[53] The effects of maternal LTBI on cytokine responses could be detected at 1 week of age but were not present later, as previously observed in South Africa.[52] A greater effect was seen when comparing Ugandan infants born to mothers with or without a BCG scar.[54] A BCG scar indicated that the individual had been BCG-vaccinated; however, the lack of a detectable scar did not guarantee that an individual had not been vaccinated, as scars can fade or be lost with time.[55] BCG-vaccinated infants born to mothers with BCG scars did show greater cytokine responses including IFNγ.[54] This may indicate some long-term effects of BCG vaccination in the mother that influences her offspring, or that those individuals who have the largest or most long-lasting scars[55] pass on the ability to respond well to BCG vaccination. There may be many other factors that influence how an infant responds to BCG vaccination including the maternal microbiome and the immaturity and subsequent rate of maturation of the infant immune system,[46] although other factors such as delaying BCG vaccination have not been shown to have a consistent enhancement in BCG immunogenicity.[10,56–58]

DOES VARIABILITY IN IMMUNE RESPONSES AND MEASURED BIOMARKERS MATTER?

The variable protection observed with BCG vaccination in adolescents and adults has been documented in a series of reviews and metaanalyses[2,4] with the strongest protection observed at higher latitudes. Such geographic variability has not been documented for the protective efficacy of BCG vaccination against the disseminated forms of TB in infants and young children. Data have been reported from South America (Brazil, Argentina), India, Indonesia, and Papua New Guinea, but no African studies were available to include.[1,3] Most of the studies reporting BCG-induced biomarkers in African infants have been too small to include progression to disease as an outcome,[10,12,53,54,59] with the exception of the studies from the Worcester BCG-vaccinated infant cohort.[20,24] It is therefore currently unclear whether the documented geographic variations in innate and acquired immunity influence protection against TB.[60]

Often, it is the balance of immune mediators or cell types that may be most critical in protection rather than the absolute quantity of a particular analyte. Here, the availability of multiplex bead array technology has provided interesting additional data. The BCG-vaccinated Malawian infants previously discussed who had reduced IFNγ responses to PPD at 3 or 12 months post-BCG vaccination[12] were found to have greater amounts of type 2 and immunoregulatory cytokines than their UK counterparts.[61] In adults, such a skewing toward the production of cytokines such as IL-4, IL-5, IL-13, or regulatory cytokines such as IL-10 might be assumed to be the result of intestinal helminths, as helminth infections have been shown to alter the cytokine balance. However, the Malawian infants in the Lalor study[61] were not found to be infected with helminths, with only a couple of infected children detected by 12 months of age from a cohort of > 500 infants. A major mother and baby study in Uganda in which mothers were given anthelminthic treatment during pregnancy showed that treatment failed to enhance BCG-induced IFNγ responses.[62,63] HIV infection will also modulate the immune responses detected, but again in most of the reported studies, HIV screening did not detect evidence of infection. Similarly, comorbidity with diabetes might impact on the efficacy of BCG vaccination as a host-directed therapy.

These findings do however indicate that, when used as an immunomodulatory treatment for autoimmune diseases, the efficacy of BCG vaccination may vary depending on coinfections and comorbidity.

CONCLUSIONS

The BCG vaccine is widely used and, although much research aims to develop an improved vaccine against TB, it is likely that the existing BCG vaccines will continue to be given to the world's infants for the foreseeable future. There is still far too much that we do not understand about how BCG works.[64] Simplistic assumptions involving induction of antigen-specific T cells making IFNγ that would induce macrophage activation with subsequent antimycobacterial effects have proved hard to confirm through direct biomarker measurement. We need to understand whether the same protective mechanisms operate in infants and children as in adults. We need far greater insights into the underlying causes of the variability in both protective efficacy and biomarker induction resulting from BCG vaccination in different settings. The greater knowledge obtained from gene expression analyses and dissection of epigenetic effects will be very valuable, as these effects may also impact the efficacy of new TB vaccines. The effects of geographical setting, maternal influences, genetics and epigenetics, coinfections, and comorbidities require better understanding, as they may influence not only how BCG protects against TB but its potential as a host-directed therapy against autoimmune diseases.

ACKNOWLEDGMENTS

H.M. Dockrell acknowledges support as part of the EU Horizon2020 funded TBVAC2020 Consortium Grant no H2020 PHC-643381. She thanks Steven Smith and Helen Fletcher for helpful discussions and for critically reviewing the manuscript.

REFERENCES

1. Colditz GA, Brewer TF, Berkey CS, et al. Efficacy of BCG vaccine in the prevention of tuberculosis. Meta-analysis of the published literature. *JAMA.* 1994;271(9):698–702.
2. Mangtani P, Abubakar I, Ariti C, et al. Protection by BCG vaccine against tuberculosis: a systematic review of randomized controlled trials. *Clin Infect Dis.* 2014;58(4):470–480.

3. Trunz BB, Fine P, Dye C. Effect of BCG vaccination on childhood tuberculous meningitis and miliary tuberculosis worldwide: a meta-analysis and assessment of cost-effectiveness. *Lancet.* 2006;367(9517):1173–1180.

4. Fine PE.Variation in protection by BCG: implications of and for heterologous immunity. *Lancet.* 1995;346(8986):1339–1345.

5. Marinova D, Gonzalo-Asensio J, Aguilo N, Martin C. MTBVAC from discovery to clinical trials in tuberculosis-endemic countries. *Expert Rev Vaccines.* 2017;16(6): 565–576.

6. Gengenbacher M, Nieuwenhuizen NE, Kaufmann S. BCG-old workhorse, new skills. *Curr Opin Immunol.* 2017;47:8–16.

7. Fletcher HA. Sleeping beauty and the story of the bacille calmette-guerin vaccine. *MBio.* 2016;7(4):e01370-16.

8. Fletcher HA, Dockrell HM. Human biomarkers: can they help us to develop a new tuberculosis vaccine? *Future Microbiol.* 2016;11:781–787.

9. Kaufmann SHE, Dockrell HM, Drager N, et al. TBVAC2020: advancing tuberculosis vaccines from discovery to clinical development. *Front Immunol.* 2017;8:1203.

10. Marchant A, Goetghebuer T, Ota MO, et al. Newborns develop a Th1-type immune response to *Mycobacterium bovis* Bacillus Calmette-Guerin vaccination. *J Immunol.* 1999;163(4):2249–2255.

11. Black GF, Weir RE, Floyd S, et al. BCG-induced increase in interferon-gamma response to mycobacterial antigens and efficacy of BCG vaccination in Malawi and the UK: two randomised controlled studies. *Lancet.* 2002;359(9315):1393–1401.

12. Lalor MK, Ben-Smith A, Gorak-Stolinska P, et al. Population differences in immune responses to Bacille Calmette-Guerin vaccination in infancy. *J Infect Dis.* 2009;199(6):795–800.

13. Cooper AM, Dalton DK, Stewart TA, Griffin JP, Russell DG, Orme IM. Disseminated tuberculosis in interferon gamma gene-disrupted mice. *J Exp Med.* 1993;178(6):2243–2247.

14. Elias D, Akuffo H, Britton S. PPD induced *in vitro* interferon gamma production is not a reliable correlate of protection against *Mycobacterium tuberculosis. Trans R Soc Trop Med Hyg.* 2005;99(5):363–368.

15. Badell E, Nicolle F, Clark S, et al. Protection against tuberculosis induced by oral prime with *Mycobacterium bovis* BCG and intranasal subunit boost based on the vaccine candidate Ag85B-ESAT-6 does not correlate with circulating IFN-gamma producing T-cells. *Vaccine.* 2009;27(1):28–37.

16. Lewinsohn DA, Lewinsohn DM, Scriba TJ. Polyfunctional CD4(+) T cells as targets for tuberculosis vaccination. *Front Immunol.* 2017;8:1262.

17. Darrah PA, Patel DT, De Luca PM, et al. Multifunctional TH1 cells define a correlate of vaccine-mediated protection against *Leishmania major. Nat Med.* 2007;13(7):843–850.

18. Smith SG, Zelmer A, Blitz R, Fletcher HA, Dockrell HM. Polyfunctional CD4 T-cells correlate with in vitro mycobacterial growth inhibition following *Mycobacterium bovis* BCG-vaccination of infants. *Vaccine.* 2016;34(44):5298–5305.

19. Smith SG, Lalor MK, Gorak-Stolinska P, et al. *Mycobacterium tuberculosis* PPD-induced immune biomarkers measurable in vitro following BCG vaccination of UK adolescents by multiplex bead array and intracellular cytokine staining. *BMC Immunol.* 2010;11:35.

20. Hawkridge A, Hatherill M, Little F, et al. Efficacy of percutaneous versus intradermal BCG in the prevention of tuberculosis in South Africa infants: randomised trial. *Br Med J.* 2008;337:a2052.

21. Hatherill M, Hawkridge T, Zar HJ, et al. Induced sputum or gastric lavage for community-based diagnosis of childhood pulmonary tuberculosis? *Arch Dis Child.* 2009;94(3):195–201.

22. Kagina BM, Abel B, Scriba TJ, et al. Specific T cell frequency and cytokine expression profile do not correlate with protection against tuberculosis after bacillus Calmette-Guerin vaccination of newborns. *Am J Respir Crit Care Med*. 2010;182(8):1073–1079.

23. Finan C, Ota MO, Marchant A, Newport MJ. Natural variation in immune responses to neonatal *Mycobacterium bovis* Bacillus Calmette-Guerin (BCG) vaccination in a Cohort of Gambian infants. *PLoS One*. 2008;3(10):e3485.

24. Fletcher HA, Filali-Mouhim A, Nemes E, et al. Human newborn bacille Calmette-Guerin vaccination and risk of tuberculosis disease: a case-control study. *BMC Med*. 2016;14:76.

25. Fletcher HA, Snowden MA, Landry B, et al. T-cell activation is an immune correlate of risk in BCG vaccinated infants. *Nat Commun*. 2016;7:11290.

26. Tameris MD, Hatherill M, Landry BS, et al. Safety and efficacy of MVA85A, a new tuberculosis vaccine, in infants previously vaccinated with BCG: a randomised, placebo-controlled phase 2b trial. *Lancet*. 2013;381(9871):1021–1028.

27. Tanner R, O'Shea MK, Fletcher HA, McShane H. In vitro mycobacterial growth inhibition assays: a tool for the assessment of protective immunity and evaluation of tuberculosis vaccine efficacy. *Vaccine*. 2016;34(39):4656–4665.

28. Zelmer A, Tanner R, Stylianou E, et al. A new tool for tuberculosis vaccine screening: ex vivo mycobacterial growth inhibition assay indicates BCG-mediated protection in a murine model of tuberculosis. *BMC Infect Dis*. 2016;16:412.

29. Brennan MJ, Tanner R, Morris S, et al. The cross-species mycobacterial growth inhibition assay (MGIA) project, 2010-2014. *Clin Vaccine Immunol*. 2017;24. pii: e00142-17.

30. Cheon SH, Kampmann B, Hise AG, et al. Bactericidal activity in whole blood as a potential surrogate marker of immunity after vaccination against tuberculosis. *Clin Diagn Lab Immunol*. 2002;9(4):901–907.

31. Silver RF, Li Q, Boom WH, Ellner JJ. Lymphocyte-dependent inhibition of growth of virulent *Mycobacterium tuberculosis* H37Rv within human monocytes: requirement for CD4+ T cells in purified protein derivative-positive, but not in purified protein derivative-negative subjects. *J Immunol*. 1998;160(5):2408–2417.

32. Hoft DF, Worku S, Kampmann B, et al. Investigation of the relationships between immune-mediated inhibition of mycobacterial growth and other potential surrogate markers of protective *Mycobacterium tuberculosis* immunity. *J Infect Dis*. 2002;186(10):1448–1457.

33. Worku S, Hoft DF. Differential effects of control and antigen-specific T cells on intracellular mycobacterial growth. *Infect Immun*. 2003;71(4):1763–1773.

34. Kampmann B, Tena GN, Mzazi S, Eley B, Young DB, Levin M. Novel human *in vitro* system for evaluating antimycobacterial vaccines. *Infect Immun*. 2004;72(11):6401–6407.

35. Plotkin SA. Complex correlates of protection after vaccination. *Clin Infect Dis*. 2013;56(10):1458–1465.

36. Vesikari T. Rotavirus vaccination: a concise review. *Clin Microbiol Infect*. 2012;18(Suppl. 5): 57–63.

37. Wilson ME, Fineberg HV, Colditz GA. Geographic latitude and the efficacy of bacillus Calmette-Guerin vaccine. *Clin Infect Dis*. 1995;20(4):982–991.

38. Black GF, Weir RE, Chaguluka SD, et al. Gamma interferon responses induced by a panel of recombinant and purified mycobacterial antigens in healthy, non-*Mycobacterium bovis* BCG-vaccinated Malawian young adults. *Clin Diagn Lab Immunol*. 2003;10(4):602–611.

39. Black GF, Dockrell HM, Crampin AC, et al. Patterns and implications of naturally acquired immune responses to environmental and tuberculous mycobacterial antigens in northern Malawi. *J Infect Dis*. 2001;184(3):322–329.

40. Checkley AM, Wyllie DH, Scriba TJ, et al. Identification of antigens specific to non-tuberculous mycobacteria: the Mce family of proteins as a target of T cell immune responses. *PLoS One*. 2011;6(10):e26434.

41. Brandt L, Feino Cunha J, Weinreich Olsen A, et al. Failure of the *Mycobacterium bovis* BCG vaccine: some species of environmental mycobacteria block multiplication of BCG and induction of protective immunity to tuberculosis. *Infect Immun*. 2002;70(2):672–678.
42. Flaherty DK, Vesosky B, Beamer GL, Stromberg P, Turner J. Exposure to M*ycobacterium avium* can modulate established immunity against *Mycobacterium tuberculosis* infection generated by *Mycobacterium bovis* BCG vaccination. *J Leukoc Biol*. 2006;80(6):1262–1271.
43. Dopico XC, Evangelou M, Ferreira RC, et al. Widespread seasonal gene expression reveals annual differences in human immunity and physiology. *Nat Commun*. 2015;6:7000.
44. Miles DJ, van der Sande M, Crozier S, et al. Effects of antenatal and postnatal environments on CD4 T-cell responses to *Mycobacterium bovis* BCG in healthy infants in the Gambia. *Clin Vaccine Immunol*. 2008;15(6):995–1002.
45. Hur YG, Gorak-Stolinska P, Lalor MK, et al. Factors affecting immunogenicity of BCG in infants, a study in Malawi, the Gambia and the UK. *BMC Infect Dis*. 2014;4:184.
46. Kampmann B, Jones CE. Factors influencing innate immunity and vaccine responses in infancy. *Philos Trans R Soc Lond B Biol Sci*. 2015;370(1671):20140148.
47. Dominguez-Salas P, Moore SE, Baker MS, et al. Maternal nutrition at conception modulates DNA methylation of human metastable epialleles. *Nat Commun*. 2014;5:3746.
48. Kleinnijenhuis J, Quintin J, Preijers F, et al. Bacille Calmette-Guerin induces NOD2-dependent nonspecific protection from reinfection via epigenetic reprogramming of monocytes. *Proc Natl Acad Sci USA*. 2012;109(43):17537–17542.
49. Smith SG, Kleinnijenhuis J, Netea MG, Dockrell HM. Whole blood profiling of bacillus Calmette-Guerin-induced trained innate immunity in infants identifies epidermal growth factor, IL-6, platelet-derived growth factor-AB/BB, and natural killer cell activation. *Front Immunol*. 2017;8:644.
50. Kleinnijenhuis J, van Crevel R, Netea MG. Trained immunity: consequences for the heterologous effects of BCG vaccination. *Trans R Soc Trop Med Hyg*. 2015;109(1):29–35.
51. Verma D, Parasa VR, Raffetseder J, et al. Anti-mycobacterial activity correlates with altered DNA methylation pattern in immune cells from BCG-vaccinated subjects. *Sci Rep*. 2017;7(1):12305.
52. Jones CE, Hesseling AC, Tena-Coki NG, et al. The impact of HIV exposure and maternal *Mycobacterium tuberculosis* infection on infant immune responses to Bacille Calmette-Guerin vaccination. *AIDS*. 2015;29(2):155–165.
53. Mawa PA, Nkurunungi G, Egesa M, et al. The impact of maternal infection with *Mycobacterium tuberculosis* on the infant response to bacille Calmette-Guerin immunization. *Philos Trans R Soc Lond B Biol Sci*. 2015;370(1671):20140137.
54. Mawa PA, Webb EL, Filali-Mouhim A, et al. Maternal BCG scar is associated with increased infant proinflammatory immune responses. *Vaccine*. 2017;35(2):273–282.
55. Floyd S, Ponnighaus JM, Bliss L, et al. BCG scars in northern Malawi: sensitivity and repeatability of scar reading, and factors affecting scar size. *Int J Tuberc Lung Dis*. 2000;4(12):1133–1142.
56. Burl S, Adetifa UJ, Cox M, et al. Delaying bacillus Calmette-Guerin vaccination from birth to 4 1/2 months of age reduces postvaccination Th1 and IL-17 responses but leads to comparable mycobacterial responses at 9 months of age. *J Immunol*. 2010;185(4): 2620–2628.
57. Tchakoute CT, Hesseling AC, Kidzeru EB, et al. Delaying BCG vaccination until 8 weeks of age results in robust BCG-specific T-cell responses in HIV-exposed infants. *J Infect Dis*. 2015;211(3):338–346.
58. Lutwama F, Kagina BM, Wajja A, et al. Distinct T-cell responses when BCG vaccination is delayed from birth to 6 weeks of age in Ugandan infants. *J Infect Dis*. 2014;209(6):887–897.
59. Lee H, Cho SN, Kim HJ, et al. Evaluation of cell-mediated immune responses to two BCG vaccination regimes in young children in South Korea. *Vaccine*. 2011;29(38):6564–6571.

60. Dockrell HM, Smith SG, Lalor MK.Variability between countries in cytokine responses to BCG vaccination: what impact might this have on protection? *Expert Rev Vaccines*. 2012;11(2):121–124.
61. Lalor MK, Floyd S, Gorak-Stolinska P, et al. BCG vaccination induces different cytokine profiles following infant BCG vaccination in the UK and Malawi. *J Infect Dis*. 2011;204(7):1075–1085.
62. Elliott AM, Mawa PA, Webb EL, et al. Effects of maternal and infant co-infections, and of maternal immunisation, on the infant response to BCG and tetanus immunisation. *Vaccine*. 2010;29(2):247–255.
63. Webb EL, Mawa PA, Ndibazza J, et al. Effect of single-dose anthelmintic treatment during pregnancy on an infant's response to immunisation and on susceptibility to infectious diseases in infancy: a randomised, double-blind, placebo-controlled trial. *Lancet*. 2011;377(9759):52–62.
64. Moliva JI, Turner J, Torrelles JB. Immune responses to Bacillus Calmette-Guerin vaccination: why do they fail to protect against *Mycobacterium tuberculosis*? *Front Immunol*. 2017;8:407.

CHAPTER 6

The Heterologous Effects of Bacillus Calmette-Guérin (BCG) Vaccine and Trained Innate Immunity

Boris Novakovic*, Nicole L. Messina*,†, Nigel Curtis*,†,‡
*Cancer & Disease Epigenetics and Infectious Diseases & Microbiology Research Groups, Murdoch Children's Research Institute, Parkville, VIC, Australia
†Department of Paediatrics, The University of Melbourne, Parkville, VIC, Australia
‡Infectious Diseases Unit, The Royal Children's Hospital Melbourne, Parkville, VIC, Australia

Contents

THE BCG VACCINE

Bacillus Calmette-Guérin (BCG) is a live-attenuated strain of *Mycobacterium bovis* that protects against mycobacterial diseases, including tuberculosis (TB) and leprosy.[1,2] BCG has more than 80% protective efficacy against the

The Value of BCG and TNF in Autoimmunity
https://doi.org/10.1016/B978-0-12-814603-3.00006-9

severe forms of TB (such as meningitis and disseminated disease) that affect infants and children, but the vaccine has limited efficacy, ranging from 0% to 80% against pulmonary TB in adults.[3] The World Health Organization (WHO) recommends BCG vaccination at birth for all infants in TB-endemic regions, with the aim of reducing TB deaths by 95% by 2035.[4] Given to more than 120 million infants globally each year, BCG is one of the most widely used vaccines. Despite the use of BCG for almost a century, TB continues to cause more than 1 million deaths each year, and it is estimated that one-third of the population is infected with the causative pathogen *Mycobacterium tuberculosis*.

NONSPECIFIC (HETEROLOGOUS) EFFECTS OF BCG VACCINE

There is a large and rapidly expanding body of evidence that BCG also has beneficial "nonspecific" (heterologous) effects greater than protection against TB alone. These heterologous effects of BCG were first reported in Sweden in 1931, just 3 years after the introduction of the vaccine in that country.[5] Since then, BCG vaccination has been associated with protection of both children and adults against a multitude of diseases including infections, immune-mediated diseases and cancer.

Human Epidemiological Studies

The earliest indication of the beneficial heterologous effects of BCG in humans came from the observation that BCG vaccination reduced childhood mortality to a greater extent than could be attributed to prevention of TB deaths alone.[5] An early observational study in Sweden found that, for an infant population in which TB accounted for approximately 2% of deaths, BCG-vaccinated infants had reduced mortality rates of 6.6% compared with 22% in the non–BCG-vaccinated infants.[5] In contrast, early clinical trials among Native Indian populations in the United States and Canada found no effect of BCG vaccination on mortality not associated with TB.[6–8] However, these trials were considered at moderate risk for bias.[9]

Further epidemiological studies in high mortality settings have also found reduced all-cause infant mortality as a result of BCG vaccination at birth.[10–13] The findings of these observational trials encouraged future clinical trials. A randomized controlled trial (RCT) involving a total of 2343 low-birth-weight newborns in Guinea-Bissau reported considerable reduced all-cause mortality in infants vaccinated with BCG at birth compared with those for whom BCG vaccination was delayed.[14] This protection against all-cause mortality was dramatic and rapid; neonatal BCG vaccination reduced infant deaths at 1 month of age by 45% (11%–67%), and the effects were evident as early as 3 days after BCG vaccination.[14,15]

The accumulating evidence for protection against all-cause mortality prompted the WHO to commission a review of studies assessing the impact of BCG on childhood mortality. The meta-analysis included five clinical trials and nine observations studies, eight of which were cohort studies and one case control study. The meta-analysis found that BCG vaccination reduces all-cause mortality in children under 5 years of age by 30% in the clinical trials and by 53% in the observation studies.[9]

Interestingly, a more recently published study, which amalgamated the data from 6583 children in three RCTs of neonatal BCG vaccination in Guinea-Bissau, found differential effects of age and BCG on all-cause mortality between girls and boys in the first month of life.[14,16] Specifically, BCG-vaccinated boys had a threefold lower risk of all-cause mortality in the first week of life compared with non–BCG-vaccinated boys. However, this protective effect in boys was no longer evident at 2 to 4 weeks of age. In contrast, BCG vaccination reduced all-cause mortality in girls at 2 to 4 weeks of age but had no effect in the first week of life.[16] This differential effect may be related to the greater than twofold increased all-cause mortality in boys compared with girls in the first week of life.[16]

BCG and Infectious Diseases

Few of the studies that have assessed the protection against all-cause mortality by BCG vaccination have collected cause of death data, but the reduced mortality has been attributed to lower rates of sepsis, respiratory tract infections, and diarrhea.[17–19]

The protection afforded by BCG vaccination against infections in humans is consistent with the plethora of animal studies showing that BCG protects against a wide range of pathogens including bacteria (such as *Shigella flexneri*),[20] viruses (such as vaccinia virus),[21] fungi (such as *Candida albicans*),[22] and protozoa (such as *Plasmodium* spp.).[23,24]

A study of acute lower respiratory tract infections in 386 infants in Guinea-Bissau found a greater than twofold increased risk of acute lower respiratory tract infections in infants who were not BCG vaccinated and a 1.5-fold increased risk for BCG-vaccinated infants who did not develop a BCG scar compared with scar-positive BCG-vaccinated infants.[25] Interestingly, in this study, the effect of BCG was stronger in girls than in boys. The ability of BCG vaccine to protect against infections other than TB has also been reported in countries with low infant mortality. Two large epidemiological studies have shown that BCG vaccination is associated with protection against respiratory tract infections. The first was a 25-year population-based retrospective analysis of more than 40,000 children with acute lower respiratory tract infection from 33 countries undertaken by Johns Hopkins Bloomberg School of Public Health. This study found that, for children under 5 years of age, BCG vaccination reduced the risk of acute lower respiratory tract infections by 17% to 37%.[26] The second study, a retrospective epidemiological study of 464,611 pediatric hospitalizations in Spain, reported a 41% lower risk of serious respiratory infection and 53% lower risk of sepsis not related to TB for BCG-vaccinated children.[27] A recent epidemiological study of 19,363 children from Greenland with 2069 hospitalizations due to infectious diseases reported that BCG vaccination afforded no protection against infections (any infection or respiratory tract infections) requiring hospitalization in children 3 months to 3 years of age.[28] However, this study did find evidence for protection against infection by BCG vaccination in the first 3 months of life,[29] consistent with the hypothesis that the beneficial heterologous effects of BCG are negated by subsequent nonlive vaccines.[30,31]

A recent RCT in Denmark investigating the effect of neonatal BCG vaccination on multiple infant health outcomes also found that BCG vaccination reduced acute lower respiratory tract infections in the first 3 months of life. However, this effect was restricted to infants whose mothers were also BCG vaccinated and was not apparent in older children.[32] This is an interesting observation in light of the fact that the majority of the previous studies of BCG's protection against nonmycobacterial infections have been in countries where maternal BCG vaccination rates are likely high.

BCG and Cancer

In addition to protecting against infections, there is evidence that BCG protects against malignancies. Several studies in the 1970s reported an up to 50% reduction in leukemia deaths among BCG-vaccinated children.[33] Despite early promise, controlled trials during this same era failed to confirm this effect.[33] Recently, a meta-analysis of 12 studies published from 1962 to 2007 concluded that BCG-vaccinated children had a 27% reduced risk of leukemia.[34] BCG has also been associated with protection against melanoma. A case-control study recently suggested that the risk of melanoma development was decreased by 33% in patients vaccinated with BCG.[35] Importantly, vaccination in early life was associated with better survival after diagnosis of melanoma.[36] It has been hypothesized that this protective effect of BCG against leukemia and melanoma, the former linked to suboptimal immune priming,[37,38] results from the beneficial effect of BCG on immune maturation in newborns.[39]

Given its potent immunomodulatory effects, BCG has also been trialed as an immunotherapeutic and cancer vaccine adjuvant for multiple types of cancer including melanoma, leukemia, breast cancer, bladder cancer, and lung cancer. RCTs have failed to demonstrate efficacy of BCG in the treatment of many of these cancer types, with the exception of bladder cancer. Intravesical BCG treatment for superficial bladder cancer was approved by the TGA in the United States in 1990 and remains the gold standard treatment worldwide for this malignancy, providing an average 27% reduction in the risk of progression.[40]

BCG and Allergy

The immunomodulatory effects of BCG vaccination have been associated with decreased severity of asthma,[41] allergy, and eczema.[42] Recent studies also suggest a potential role for BCG to reduce progression of type I diabetes and multiple sclerosis.[43,44] Due to the declining prevalence of TB, the routine administration of BCG was stopped in a number of industrialized countries in the mid-1980s. This was notably coincident, but not causally verified, to a subsequent increase in childhood allergic disease.

The immunomodulatory effects of BCG vaccination are proposed to involve the promotion of T helper (Th)1 function and inhibition of Th2 responses.[39] Allergic disease in contrast are associated with increased Th2 activity.[45] Consequently, there is considerable interest in whether immunization with BCG in infancy, by skewing host immunity from an early age away from a "Th2 allergic pathway" while promoting a "Th1 pathway," might reduce the prevalence of allergic disorders in high-income countries (Fig. 6.1). Experimental evidence from animal models and epidemiological data in humans support this hypothesis.

In mice, BCG immunization diminishes allergic sensitization and the development of increased airway reactivity.[46] Furthermore, administration of *Mycobacterium vaccae* inhibits an established allergic response to ovalbumin in mice[47] and, together with *M. bovis* at birth, decreases immunoglobulin (Ig) E serum levels in sensitized mice.[48] *M. vaccae* also prevents the histological changes usually observed in the lungs in chronic asthma.[49]

In humans, multiple observational studies report protection against allergic diseases by BCG vaccination. However, due to high heterogeneity

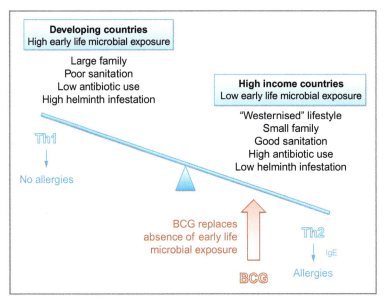

Fig. 6.1 A hypothetical model for a beneficial role of BCG in allergies. In this model, BCG acts as an early life microbial exposure, skewing immune development from Th2 to Th1 function.

in study design and populations, meta-analyses studies have failed to reach reliable conclusions on this.[41,45,50] A major limitation in this field is the dearth of RCTs of adequate size to test the effect of neonatal BCG on allergies. At the time of the meta-analysis study, there was only one RCT of BCG vaccine given at birth to prevent the development of allergic disease. This study, although small with only 121 participants, found that BCG vaccination reduced eczema medication use and clinically assessed eczema by 42% and 28%, respectively.[51] There have subsequently been two large RCTs of BCG, one based in Copenhagen, Denmark (Calmette study[32]), and the other in Melbourne, Australia (The Melbourne Infant Study: BCG for Allergy and Infection Reduction; MIS BAIR). Although the findings of the MIS BAIR study are yet to be published, similar to the previous RCT, the Calmette study found a significant reduction in clinically diagnosed eczema,[52] although no BCG effect was found on childhood food allergy.[53]

There have also been numerous observational studies investigating the apparent protective effect of BCG vaccination on the development of asthma. For example, in a study in Japanese schoolchildren, those with a positive tuberculin skin test (indicating exposure to BCG) had a lower incidence of asthma, lower serum IgE levels, and Th1-type cytokine profiles. Similarly, a small clinical trial in Mexico, which used alternate allocation of only 67 subjects, found significant immunological changes associated with BCG, although the trial was inadequately powered to detect an effect of BCG on the measured clinical outcomes.[54] In this study, levels of IgE and interleukin (IL)-4 (markers of a Th2 response) increased in the control group but did not change in the BCG group, whereas interferon (IFN)-γ (a marker of Th1 response) decreased in the control group but did not change in the BCG group, supporting the hypothesis that BCG primes the immune response away from an allergic pathway. Overall, although limited data is available, two meta-analysis studies concluded that BCG vaccination reduces the risk of childhood asthma by 14% to 27%.[41,50]

BCG AND IMMUNOMODULATION

Consistent with the beneficial heterologous effects of BCG on health outcomes, the heterologous immunological effects of BCG vaccination occur rapidly (within 1 week of vaccination[55]) and can persist for at least 5 years.[22,56] This indicates that the responsible mechanisms are both fast-acting and long-lasting.

Cytokine Studies

Multiple studies in both infants and adults show that BCG vaccination alters cytokine responses to Toll-like receptor (TLR) agonists, such as peptidoglycan (TLR2) (S)-(2,3-bis (palmitoyloxy)-(2-RS)-propyl)-N-palmitoyl-(R)-Cys-(S)-Ser-(S)-Lys4OH, trihydrochloride (PAMcys3; TLR1/2), R848 (TLR7/8), and nonmycobacterial pathogens, such as *C. albicans, S. aureus,* and *Listeria monocytogenes.*[22,55–58] In response to heterologous stimuli, BCG alters production of cytokines associated with inflammation, such as tumor necrosis factor (TNF)-α and IL-1β; Th1 responses, such as IL12-p40 and IFN-γ; Th-17 responses, such as IL-17; and immunosuppression, such as IL-10 and IL-1ra.[22,55–58] In addition, BCG alters the production of chemokines, such as IL-8 (CXCL-8), monocyte chemotactic protein 1 (MCP)-1 (CCL-2), and macrophage inflammatory protein (MIP)-1α (CCL-3); and growth factors, such as epidermal growth factor (EGF) and platelet-derived growth factor (PDGF).[55,57] BCG differentially alters the production of these cytokines, chemokines, and growth factors in response to the various heterologous stimuli, however, the mechanisms governing this have yet to be elucidated.

The two recent RCTs assessing the effects of neonatal BCG vaccination on health outcomes have both assessed cytokine responses to heterologous antigens with varying results. The Danish Calmette study found no BCG-induced changes in cytokine production following stimulation with five heterologous antigens 4 days after randomization.[59] However, 3 months after randomization, samples from BCG-vaccinated infants had decreased production of two cytokines (IL-10 and IL-17) in response to *C. albicans* stimulation.[59] In the Australian MIS BAIR study, BCG vaccination reduced cytokine and chemokine production following stimulation with 6 of 12 heterologous antigens tested 7 days after randomization.[55] The disparate findings for early cytokine responses may be due to multiple experimental factors, including differences in sampling timing (4 days compared with 7 days postrandomization), stimulation times (24 and 96 h compared with 20 h), and concomitant vaccines (none compared with hepatitis B), as well as the choice of cytokines and chemokines assessed.

Notably, although both studies reported an effect of age at BCG vaccination on early cytokine responses to heterologous antigens, these effects were in opposite directions. The Calmette study found increased cytokine responses for infants randomized to BCG at least 2 days after birth.[59] In contrast, the MIS BAIR study found that BCG vaccination at least 2 days after birth was associated with a stronger attenuation of cytokine responses than early BCG vaccination.[55] It will be of interest in the future to determine if the early differences in cytokine response correlate with the effect of BCG on health outcomes in these clinical trials.

Vaccine Response Studies

BCG also influences the host's response to other vaccines.[60,61] Studies of humeral vaccine responses after infant BCG vaccination show that BCG regulates antibody response to hepatitis B, polio, tetanus, Hib, and pneumococcal vaccines.[58,60,62,63] Interestingly, BCG administered at the time of primary immunization markedly increases the cellular responses to hepatitis B, while having no effect or decreasing humoural responses.[60,62] In adults, BCG vaccination increases humoural responses to influenza vaccine and decreases viral load following vaccination with yellow-fever vaccine, however, it has no effect on specific cytokine responses to either of these vaccines.[64,65]

Immunological Mechanisms

Two types of immunological mechanisms have been suggested to mediate the heterologous effects of BCG vaccination. First, CD4$^+$ and CD8$^+$

memory cells can be activated in an antigen-independent manner (e.g., by cytokines stimulated by a secondary infection), a process called heterologous immunity.[21,66] Second, a growing area of study suggests that some of the beneficial heterologous effects of BCG are mediated by cells of the innate immune system through a process termed "innate immune memory" or trained immunity (TRIM).

Adaptive Immune Cells

It is postulated that the beneficial heterologous effects of BCG on human health outcomes, particularly for immune-mediated diseases, are due at least in part to BCG promoting Th1 polarization of the developing infant immune system.[39] However, reports of the impact of BCG on adaptive immune responses and their contribution to the beneficial heterologous effects of BCG are inconsistent. The impact of BCG vaccination on adaptive immune responses to unrelated pathogens has primarily been assessed in animal models, and the results have been variable.[24] In a murine model of candidiasis, BCG protected mice which lack T- and B-cell responses (Rag1-deficient mice) against lethal candidiasis, indicating that adaptive immune responses were dispensable for BCG-mediated protection.[22] In contrast, in a model of BCG-induced protection from malaria lethality, depletion of $CD8^+$ T cells prior to infection abrogated the protective effect of BCG.[23]

In humans, one study has assessed the effect of BCG vaccination on cytokine responses of T cells. After stimulation of PBMCs with the antigen-independent stimulus PMA/ionomycin, there was a significant increase in the proportion of antigen-experienced ($CD45RO^+$) $CD4^+$ T cells producing IFN-γ and TNF-α in samples from BCG-vaccinated infants compared with non-BCG-vaccinated infants.[63] Studies in humans report varying effects of BCG vaccination on the frequency of T cell subpopulations.[56,58,63,67] Studies of T-cell populations in BCG-vaccinated infants compared with non-BCG-vaccinated infants, and before and after BCG vaccination of adults, show no effect of BCG on total numbers of $CD4^+$, $CD8^+$, and $CD3^+$ populations, although one study did find decreased proportions of $CD8^+$ T cells among $CD3^+$ T cells 2 weeks to 1 year after BCG vaccination.[56,67] Similarly, an earlier study found that, although BCG did not alter total T-cell receptor (TCR)-expressing populations, 2 months after BCG vaccination, numbers of $\alpha\beta$ T cells significantly decreased while numbers of $\gamma\delta$ T cells increased.[68] Notably, however, a study assessing T-cell proliferation responses found that BCG vaccination also increased proliferation responses of $CD4^+$, $CD8^+$, and $\gamma\delta$ T cells to mycobacterial antigens, and proliferation in response to tetanus toxoid.[69] These studies indicate that BCG can directly or indirectly (e.g., through changes in cytokine production by other immune cells) impact T cells.

Innate Immune Cells

Although the endurance of the beneficial heterologous effects of BCG (months to years) suggests involvement of adaptive immune cells, the rapid (as early as 3 days postvaccination) impact on infant mortality[15] and cytokine responses,[55] as well as the potential effects of BCG on a broad range of health outcomes, support the involvement of innate immune cells. A series of elegant in vitro and in vivo studies (to be described in detail later) have shown that BCG directly induces long-lasting changes to innate immune cells. These studies show that BCG exposure, either by vaccination or in vitro stimulation, increases subsequent monocyte cytokine (IL-6 and TNF-α) responses to unrelated pathogens and increases monocyte TLR4 receptor expression.[22] BCG vaccination also increases NK cell production of the proinflammatory cytokines TNF-α and IL-1β in response to heterologous antigen (*C. albicans* or *S. aureus*) stimulation.[70] A recent study of BCG vaccination in infants also found greater NK cell activation in whole blood samples from BCG-vaccinated infants stimulated with TLR 1/2-agonist PAMcys3 compared with non–BCG-vaccinated infants.[57] Importantly, these effects of BCG on innate immune cells are long-lasting and persist for at least 1 year after vaccination.[56,70] As early responders in immune responses, and given the critical links between the innate and adaptive immune systems, the effects of BCG on innate immune cells likely contributes to BCG-induced changes in adaptive immune responses.

TRAINED INNATE IMMUNITY

The concept that the innate immune system lacks capacity for memory is being questioned by a rapidly growing body of work.[71] The phenomenon of "innate immune memory" involves priming of innate immune cells, such as monocytes, by exposure to microbe-associated molecular patterns (MAMPs) during their time in the circulation or in a resident tissue.[72] In this respect, exposure of monocytes to high bacterial burden results in a subdued response to future infection and represents one extreme in a spectrum of innate immune memory.[71] In contrast, TRIM can be induced by exposure to certain vaccines, bacterial components, or metabolites, and results in a state characterized by increased proinflammatory responses to secondary unrelated infections.[73] Unlike adaptive immune memory, which is antigen-specific and depends on genetic rearrangement, TRIM is non-specific and is mediated by epigenetic mechanisms. The concept of TRIM was first proposed to explain the increased cytokine responses to subsequent bacterial and fungal exposure in BCG-vaccinated individuals.[22] Further studies showed that exposure to *C. albicans*, and specifically *C. albicans* cell wall component β-glucan, induces TRIM in mouse and human monocytes through the Dectin-1 receptor pathway.[73]

Immunometabolic Reprogramming in Trained Immunity

A major component of TRIM is a switch from oxidative phosphorylation to glycolysis, also known as the Warburg effect.[71,74] β-Glucan induces the expression of many citric acid (tricarboxylic acid, TCA) cycle genes.[75–77] Interestingly, monocyte tolerance induced by high level LPS in vitro,[77] or high bacterial burden in sepsis patients,[76] is associated with a downregulation of metabolism. Both in vitro LPS-induced and sepsis-induced tolerance can be partially reversed by reactivation of metabolism by TRIM stimuli, such as B-glucan or IFN-γ.[76,77] The centrality of the TCA cycle in TRIM is underlined by studies showing that TRIM can be induced by treating monocytes with metabolites from the TCA cycle alone, including fumarate[75] and mevalonate.[78] Interestingly itaconate, which is strongly induced in inflammation and associated with tolerance in monocytes, represses both fumarate and succinate accumulation.[79]

Epigenetic/Chromatin Reprogramming in Trained Immunity

The term "epigenetics" refers to the study of molecular interactions that influence chromosome structure and gene activity. Epigenetic mechanisms encompass covalent modifications of DNA, such as DNA methylation and posttranslational modifications of histone tails that protrude from the nucleosome, around which DNA is coiled. These modifications can be "written," "erased," and "read" by specific nuclear proteins, and this determines gene activity. These modifications occur in gene promoters, where mRNA transcription starts, and enhancers, distal cis-regulatory genomic regions that tune promoter activity and thus determine cellular phenotype. The erasure or establishment of activity at specific regulatory genomic elements is essential for monocyte differentiation[80,81] and response to exogenous stimuli.[77,82]

Monocytes and macrophages are innate immune cells that play an important role in the pathophysiology of sepsis and inflammation.[71] Differentiation of human monocytes to macrophages is associated with large-scale epigenetic and transcriptional changes that underlie the change to a phagocytic phenotype. Until recently, it was assumed that macrophage responses to infection were restricted to their primed (histone H3, Lysine-4, monomethylation; H3K4me1) or active (H3K4me1/histone H3, Lysine-27, acetylation; H3K27ac) chromatin state at gene-enhancer repertoires, largely marked by the binding of the E26 transformation-specific (ETS)-domain transcription factor PU.1 (also known as Spi-1 proto-oncogene).[83] However, an in vitro study by Ostuni et al. found that, when exposed to LPS, mouse macrophages also accumulate H3K27ac at distal gene regions not marked by H3K4me1. These have been termed "latent" enhancers. After removal of the stimulus, these regions lost H3K27ac but retained the longer half-life H3K4me1 mark, resulting in faster H3K27ac accumulation the second time cells were exposed to LPS.[82] The ability of fully differentiated cells to gain new distal gene regulatory chromatin elements, specified by distinct histone modification profiles, is novel, suggesting that exogenous signals from the environment can shape the phenotype of terminally differentiated cells and influence their response to future exposure.

TRIM is largely regulated at the level of chromatin modifications, as well as shifts in cellular metabolism.[71] In the most well-described model of TRIM, brief exposure of adult human monocytes to high levels of LPS, or to β-glucan, induces immunological tolerance or immunological training, respectively, in the absence of cell division.[81] Tolerance and TRIM are each associated with specific epigenetic and transcriptional reprogramming at the level of both histone modifications and DNA methylation.[81,84] Importantly, several of the induced epigenetic marks associated with LPS-induced tolerance are reversible by β-glucan exposure ex vivo.[77] This reversal is associated with re-establishment of steady-state levels of H3K27ac at specific gene promoters and enhancers in adult human macrophages.[77] This finding suggests that TRIM can be used to carefully modulate innate immunity with the potential to develop novel immunomodulatory treatments for a range of associated inflammatory diseases.

As previously discussed, β-glucan-associated epigenetic remodeling of macrophages involves the activation of genes involved in the TCA cycle and cholesterol metabolism, and interestingly TRIM can be induced by exposure to single specific metabolites, such as fumarate and mevalonate.[75,78] Using H3K27ac whole genome chromatin immunoprecipitation linked to deep DNA sequencing (ChIP-seq), it has been shown that fumarate and mevalonate exposure induces changes in histone modifications at proinflammatory genes in adult monocytes.[71,75] The ability of different

TRIM-inducing stimuli to improve immune function in infant mono-cytes suggests the opportunity for interventions to influence susceptibility to infection and allergy.

EVIDENCE FOR BCG-INDUCED TRAINED IMMUNITY

TRIM is a complex immunometabolic process involving reprogram-ming at several levels of the cell, including chromatin, energy production, phagocytosis, and cytokine release machinery. Although the gold-standard measure of TRIM is enhanced release of cytokines, a phenomenon shared by monocytes trained by different stimuli, as yet no single common chro-matin signature has been found for the different TRIM-inducing stimuli. Therefore, it is likely that TRIM can be induced by several pathways, which modify shared cellular processes, leading to a general hyperinflammatory phenotype. In this sense, the ability of BCG to induce TRIM in human monocytes has been shown both in vivo and ex vivo.[22,85]

In Vivo Experiments

In the first proof-of-principle clinical trial of BCG vaccination-induced TRIM, Arts et al. showed that BCG-trained monocytes contributed to faster clearance of a viral infection, modeled using the yellow fever vac-cine.[65] In the trial, 30 individuals were assigned to two groups: BCG vac-cination or placebo, followed by the yellow fever vaccine 1 month later. At 5 days postyellow fever vaccination, the BCG-vaccinated group showed lower levels of viral DNA in the blood, as well as an associated higher level of IL-1β. Given the association of elevated IL-1β with TRIM, the investi-gators could conclude that TRIM-associated cytokines are involved in this process. The investigators further showed that SNPs in the IL-1β gene affect the induction of TRIM, indicating a circumstantial link between BCG vac-cination, IL-1β elevation, and TRIM in vivo.[65] This study confirmed earlier reports of BCG-induced TRIM in human monocytes in vivo,[22,56] which showed that circulating monocytes from BCG-vaccinated individuals pro-duced higher levels of IL-1β, as well as TNF-α and IL-6. NOD2 and IFN-γ signaling were both found to be important in the establishment of BCG-induced TRIM in vivo. The increased production of IFN-γ in response to unrelated MAMPs, such as C. albicans and S. aureus, was found to last up to 1 year following BCG vaccination.[56] Considering that monocytes only spend a few days in the circulation, this finding suggests that trained monocytes continue to be produced by precursors in the bone marrow long after BCG exposure (Fig. 6.2A). A recent study by Kaufmann et al.[86] provides a mechanism for BCG-induced long-term memory in monocytes by showing that BCG remodels the hematopoietic precursors in mouse bone marrow and skews them toward myeloid cell production in favor of lymphoid cells.

In Vitro Data

The in vitro monocyte-to-macrophage differentiation model has been important in uncovering the epigenetic, metabolic, and immunological processes involved in the establishment of TRIM.[81,87] Using this model, monocytes were exposed to the BCG Denmark vaccine for 24 h, and then allowed to differentiate for 6 days. The resulting macrophages produced higher levels of TNF-α and IL-6 when exposed to LPS, and showed up-regulation of mTOR, similarly to β-glucan-trained macrophages. However, unlike β-glucan training, which induced the Warburg effect, BCG-trained macrophages showed upregulation of both glycolysis and oxidative phosphorylation (Fig. 6.2B).[85] This indicates that BCG-induced TRIM involves metabolic reprogramming that is not exactly paralleled in β-glucan-induced TRIM.

EPIGENETIC REPROGRAMMING OF MONOCYTES BY BCG

Ex vivo BCG exposure was associated with an increase in the active histone mark H3K4me3 at the promoters of TNF-α and IL-6,[22] with an associated loss of the repressive histone mark H3K9me3 signal, indicative of increased activity at the promoter region (Fig. 6.2). However, this reprogramming is observed in macrophages directly exposed to BCG in vitro. The heterologous effects of BCG can be observed 5 years following vaccination,[88] and this long-term epigenetic memory cannot be tested in vitro. In the previously mentioned clinical trial of BCG, Arts et al.[65] showed that monocytes extracted from individuals 1 month after BCG vaccination had H3K27ac changes, yet gene expression changes were not present. This study was underpowered, however, with only seven donors used in the analysis and should be explored in a larger cohort. Secondly, this study only explored epigenetic changes up to 1 month following BCG vaccination, and it is yet to be tested if these epigenetic changes persist for longer. If such long-term epigenetic memory can be detected, it is most likely to be in the form of DNA methylation, a covalent epigenetic mark directly added to cytosines, in a cytosine-guanine (CpG) context. As DNA methylation is more stable

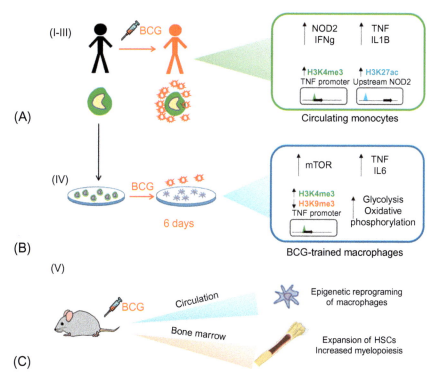

Fig. 6.2 BCG-induced TRIM. (A) Circulating monocytes from healthy volunteers vaccinated with BCG showed increased NOD2 and IFN-γ signaling,[22] increased release of TRIM cytokines such as IL-1β and TNF-α, as well as the accumulation of active histone marks, H3K4me3 and H3K27ac, at the promoter of TNF-α and upstream of the NOD2 gene, respectively.[65] (B) In vitro exposure of human monocytes to BCG-induced TRIM in macrophages, with higher release of IL-6 and TNFα, increase in both glycolysis and oxidative phosphorylation (i.e., a process different to the Warburg effect observed in β-glucan training), and accumulation of the active histone mark H3K4me3 and decrease in the repressive histone mark H3K9me3 at the promoter of TNF.[85] (C) BCG vaccination of mice resulted in epigenetic and transcriptional reprogramming of macrophages and induced the expansion of hematopoietic stem cells in the bone marrow, skewing toward the production of myeloid cells.[86]

than histone modifications, it would be the mark most likely to persist a year after BCG exposure.[3] DNA methylation has been shown to contribute to the development of human cytomegalovirus (HCMV)-induced "adaptive" NK cells.[89] To date, a single study sought to explore the effect of BCG on genome-wide DNA methylation, albeit using PBMCs and not a pure population of cells.[90] This study found that BCG vaccination altered CpG methylation at multiple sites in a T cell/monocyte-enriched population and in NK cells, however, the relationship between these changes and heterologous BCG responses was not investigated.[90] In mice, BCG vaccination reprogrammed HSCs to produce epigenetically and transcriptionally remodeled macrophages, suggesting that, in addition to circulating monocytes, BCG exposure-associated epigenetic change can potentially persist for long periods in tissue-specific macrophages.[86]

OUTSTANDING QUESTIONS AND FUTURE DIRECTIONS

In this chapter, we explored the epidemiological and experimental evidence for heterologous effects of the BCG vaccine and make the case that trained innate immunity plays an important role in this process. The last few months alone have seen several exciting experimental studies on the effect of BCG on TRIM,[65,86] as well as early reports from two large BCG clinical trials in developed countries (Calmette study and MIS BAIR), indicating that there is substantial interest in this field and more evidence to come. There are multiple questions that remain unanswered: Which immune cells contribute to the heterologous effects of BCG? How long does BCG-induced TRIM last? Does it last as long as the heterologous effects observed in epidemiological studies? Is BCG-induced TRIM mediated by hematopoietic precursor remodeling only, or do tissue-specific macrophages play a role? The availability of modern molecular profiling techniques such as single-cell RNA-seq for gene expression analysis and low input chromatin and proteomic analysis methods will allow the study of hard-to-get and low abundance cells, such as progenitor cells in the bone marrow and tissue specific macrophages. Questions also remain regarding the effects of BCG in health outcomes: What effect does BCG have in developed countries? Is it beneficial or detrimental for allergy and other autoimmune diseases that are on the rise in these countries? Do different BCG strains have different effects on TRIM, like they do on adaptive immune memory? So far, in vivo and in vitro human studies have used the BCG Denmark strain, whereas several different strains of BCG are currently in use worldwide. In conclusion, understanding the exact mechanisms involved in BCG-induced heterologous effects, complex as they may be, is paramount for current vaccine strategies and future vaccine design.

REFERENCES

1. Zumla A, Raviglione M, Hafner R, von Reyn CF. Tuberculosis. *N Engl J Med.* 2013;368:745–755.
2. Colditz GA, et al. Efficacy of BCG vaccine in the prevention of tuberculosis. Meta-analysis of the published literature. *JAMA.* 1994;271:698–702.

3. Mangtani P, et al. Protection by BCG vaccine against tuberculosis: a systematic review of randomized controlled trials. *Clin Infect Dis.* 2014;58:470–480.
4. WHO. Implementing the end TB strategy: the essentials. In: *Implementing the End TB Strategy.* Geneva: World Health Oraganization; 2016.
5. Netea MG, van Crevel R. BCG-induced protection: effects on innate immune memory. *Semin Immunol.* 2014;26:512–517.
6. Ferguson RG, Simes AB. BCG vaccination of Indian infants in Saskatchewan. *Tubercle.* 1949;30:5–11.
7. Aronson JD. Protective vaccination against tuberculosis, with special reference to BCG vaccine. *Minn Med.* 1948;31:1336.
8. Rosenthal SR, et al. BCG vaccination in tuberculous households. *Am Rev Respir Dis.* 1961;84:690–704.
9. Higgins JP, et al. Association of BCG, DTP, and measles containing vaccines with childhood mortality: systematic review. *BMJ.* 2016;355:i5170.
10. Roth A, et al. BCG vaccination scar associated with better childhood survival in Guinea-Bissau. *Int J Epidemiol.* 2005;34:540–547.
11. Kristensen I, Aaby P, Jensen H. Routine vaccinations and child survival: follow up study in Guinea-Bissau. *West Afr BMJ.* 2000;321:1435–1438.
12. Moulton LH, et al. Evaluation of non-specific effects of infant immunizations on early infant mortality in a southern Indian population. *Tropical Med Int Health.* 2005;10:947–955.
13. Hirve S, et al. Non-specific and sex-differential effects of vaccinations on child survival in rural western India. *Vaccine.* 2012;30:7300–7308.
14. Aaby P, et al. Randomized trial of BCG vaccination at birth to low-birth-weight children: beneficial nonspecific effects in the neonatal period? *J Infect Dis.* 2011;204:245–252.
15. Biering-Sorensen S, et al. Small randomized trial among low-birth-weight children receiving bacillus Calmette-Guerin vaccination at first health center contact. *Pediatr Infect Dis J.* 2012;31:306–308.
16. Biering-Sorensen S, et al. Rapid protective effects of early BCG on neonatal mortality among low birth weight boys: observations from randomized trials. *J Infect Dis.* 2018;217:759–766.
17. Shann F. The nonspecific effects of vaccines and the expanded program on immunization. *J Infect Dis.* 2011;204:182–184.
18. Shann F. The new decade of vaccines. *Lancet.* 2012;379:25–26.
19. Goodridge HS, et al. Harnessing the beneficial heterologous effects of vaccination. *Nat Rev Immunol.* 2016;16:392–400.
20. Nakamura M, Cross WR. Susceptibility of rabbits immunized with *Mycobacterium bovis* (BCG) or *Mycobacterium phlei* to *Shigella* Keratoconjunctivitis. *Infect Immun.* 1972;6:1025.
21. Mathurin KS, Martens GW, Kornfeld H, Welsh RM. CD4 T-cell-mediated heterologous immunity between mycobacteria and poxviruses. *J Virol.* 2009;83:3528–3539.
22. Kleinnijenhuis J, et al. Bacille Calmette-Guerin induces NOD2-dependent nonspecific protection from reinfection via epigenetic reprogramming of monocytes. *Proc Natl Acad Sci USA.* 2012;109:17537–17542.
23. Parra M, et al. Molecular analysis of non-specific protection against murine malaria induced by BCG vaccination. *PLoS One.* 2013;8:e66115.
24. Freyne B, Marchant A, Curtis N. BCG-associated heterologous immunity, a historical perspective: intervention studies in animal models of infectious diseases. *Trans R Soc Trop Med Hyg.* 2015;109:287.
25. Stensballe LG, et al. Acute lower respiratory tract infections and respiratory syncytial virus in infants in Guinea-Bissau: a beneficial effect of BCG vaccination for girls community based case-control study. *Vaccine.* 2005;23:1251–1257.

26. Hollm-Delgado MG, Stuart EA, Black RE. Acute lower respiratory infection among Bacille Calmette-Guerin (BCG)-vaccinated children. *Pediatrics*. 2014;133:e73–81.
27. de Castro MJ, Pardo-Seco J, Martinon-Torres F. Nonspecific (heterologous) protection of neonatal BCG vaccination against hospitalization due to respiratory infection and sepsis. *Clin Infect Dis*. 2015;60:1611–1619.
28. Haahr S, et al. Non-specific effects of BCG vaccination on morbidity among children in Greenland: a population-based cohort study. *Int J Epidemiol*. 2016;45:2122–2130.
29. Benn CS, Sorup S. Commentary: BCG has no beneficial non-specific effects on Greenland. An answer to the wrong question? *Int J Epidemiol*. 2016;45:2131–2133.
30. Flanagan KL, et al. Heterologous ("nonspecific") and sex-differential effects of vaccines: epidemiology, clinical trials, and emerging immunologic mechanisms. *Clin Infect Dis*. 2013;57:283–289.
31. Shann F. The non-specific effects of vaccines. *Arch Dis Child*. 2010;95:662–667.
32. Kjaergaard J, et al. Nonspecific effect of BCG vaccination at birth on early childhood infections: a randomized, clinical multicenter trial. *Pediatr Res*. 2016;80:681–685.
33. Hersh EM, Gutterman JU, Mavligit GM. BCG as adjuvant immunotherapy for neoplasia. *Annu Rev Med*. 1977;28:489–515.
34. Morra ME, et al. Early vaccination protects against childhood leukemia: a systematic review and meta-analysis. *Sci Rep*. 2017;7:15986.
35. Pfahlberg A, et al. Inverse association between melanoma and previous vaccinations against tuberculosis and smallpox: results of the FEBIM study. *J Invest Dermatol*. 2002;119:570–575.
36. Kolmel KF, et al. Prior immunisation of patients with malignant melanoma with vaccinia or BCG is associated with better survival. An European Organization for Research and Treatment of Cancer cohort study on 542 patients. *Eur J Cancer*. 2005;41:118–125.
37. Grange JM, Stanford JL, Stanford CA, Kolmel KF. Vaccination strategies to reduce the risk of leukaemia and melanoma. *J R Soc Med*. 2003;96:389–392.
38. Rosenthal SR. Cancer precursors and their control by BCG. *Dev Biol Stand*. 1986;58(Pt A):401–416.
39. Marchant A, et al. Newborns develop a Th1-type immune response to Mycobacterium bovis bacillus Calmette-Guerin vaccination. *J Immunol*. 1999;163:2249–2255.
40. Sylvester RJ, van der MA, Lamm DL. Intravesical bacillus Calmette-Guerin reduces the risk of progression in patients with superficial bladder cancer: a meta-analysis of the published results of randomized clinical trials. *J Urol*. 2002;168:1964–1970.
41. El-Zein M, Parent ME, Benedetti A, Rousseau MC. Does BCG vaccination protect against the development of childhood asthma? A systematic review and meta-analysis of epidemiological studies. *Int J Epidemiol*. 2010;39:469–486.
42. Freyne B, Curtis N. Does neonatal BCG vaccination prevent allergic disease in later life? *Arch Dis Child*. 2014;99:182–184.
43. Faustman DL, et al. Proof-of-concept, randomized, controlled clinical trial of Bacillus-Calmette-Guerin for treatment of long-term type 1 diabetes. *PLoS One*. 2012;7:e41756.
44. Ristori G, et al. Effects of Bacille Calmette-Guerin after the first demyelinating event in the CNS. *Neurology*. 2014;82:41–48.
45. Rousseau M-C, Parent M-E, St-Pierre Y. Potential health effects from non-specific stimulation of the immune function in early age: the example of BCG vaccination. *Pediatr Allergy Immunol*. 2008;19:438–448.
46. Herz U, et al. BCG infection suppresses allergic sensitization and development of increased airway reactivity in an animal model. *J Allergy Clin Immunol*. 1998;102:867–874.
47. Wang CC, Rook GA. Inhibition of an established allergic response to ovalbumin in BALB/c mice by killed Mycobacterium vaccae. *Immunology*. 1998;93:307–313.

48. Tukenmez F, Bahceciler NN, Barlan IB, Basaran MM. Effect of pre-immunization by killed Mycobacterium bovis and vaccae on immunoglobulin E response in ovalbumin-sensitized newborn mice. *Pediatr Allergy Immunol.* 1999;10:107–111.
49. Ozdemir C, et al. Impact of Mycobacterium vaccae immunization on lung histopathology in a murine model of chronic asthma. *Clin Exp Allergy.* 2003;33:266–270.
50. Arnoldussen DL, Linehan M, Sheikh A. BCG vaccination and allergy: a systematic review and meta-analysis. *J Allergy Clin Immunol.* 2011;127:246–253.
51. Steenhuis TJ, et al. Bacille-Calmette-Guerin vaccination and the development of allergic disease in children: a randomized, prospective, single-blind study. *Clin Exp Allergy.* 2008;38:79–85.
52. Thostesen LM, et al. Neonatal BCG vaccination and atopic dermatitis before 13 months of age: a randomized clinical trial. *Allergy.* 2018;73:498–504.
53. Thostesen LM, et al. Neonatal BCG has no effect on allergic sensitization and suspected food allergy until 13 months. *Pediatr Allergy Immunol.* 2017;28:588–596.
54. Vargas MH, Bernal-Alcántara DA, Vaca MA, Franco-Marina F, Lascurain R. Effect of BCG vaccination in asthmatic schoolchildren. *Pediatr Allergy Immunol.* 2004;15:415–420.
55. Freyne B, et al. Neonatal BCG vaccination influences cytokine responses to toll-like receptor ligands and heterologous antigens. *J Infect Dis.* 2018;217(11):1798–1808.
56. Kleinnijenhuis J, et al. Long-lasting effects of BCG vaccination on both heterologous Th1/Th17 responses and innate trained immunity. *J Innate Immun.* 2014;6:152–158.
57. Smith SG, Kleinnijenhuis J, Netea MG, Dockrell HM. Whole blood profiling of Bacillus Calmette-Guerin-induced trained innate immunity in infants identifies epidermal growth factor, IL-6, platelet-derived growth factor-AB/BB, and natural killer cell activation. *Front Immunol.* 2017;8:644.
58. Kandasamy R, et al. Non-specific immunological effects of selected routine childhood immunisations: systematic review. *BMJ.* 2016;355:i5225.
59. Nissen TN, et al. Bacillus Calmette-Guerin vaccination at birth and in vitro cytokine responses to non-specific stimulation. A randomized clinical trial. *Eur J Clin Microbiol Infect Dis.* 2018;37:29–41.
60. Ota MO, et al. Influence of Mycobacterium bovis bacillus Calmette-Guerin on antibody and cytokine responses to human neonatal vaccination. *J Immunol.* 2002;168:919–925.
61. Roth A, et al. Effect of revaccination with BCG in early childhood on mortality: randomised trial in Guinea-Bissau. *BMJ.* 2010;340:c671.
62. Ritz N, Mui M, Balloch A, Curtis N. Non-specific effect of Bacille Calmette-Guerin vaccine on the immune response to routine immunisations. *Vaccine.* 2013;31:3098–3103.
63. Libraty DH, et al. Neonatal BCG vaccination is associated with enhanced T-helper 1 immune responses to heterologous infant vaccines. *Trials Vaccinol.* 2014;3:1–5.
64. Leentjens J, et al. BCG vaccination enhances the immunogenicity of subsequent influenza vaccination in healthy volunteers: a randomized, placebo-controlled pilot study. *J Infect Dis.* 2015;212:1930–1938.
65. Arts RJW, et al. BCG vaccination protects against experimental viral infection in humans through the induction of cytokines associated with trained immunity. *Cell Host Microbe.* 2018;23:89–100. e105.
66. Lertmemongkolchai G, Cai G, Hunter CA, Bancroft GJ. Bystander activation of CD8+ T cells contributes to the rapid production of IFN-gamma in response to bacterial pathogens. *J Immunol.* 2001;166:1097–1105.
67. Birk NM, et al. Effects of Bacillus Calmette-Guerin (BCG) vaccination at birth on T and B lymphocyte subsets: results from a clinical randomized trial. *Sci Rep.* 2017;7:12398.
68. Tastan Y, et al. Influence of Bacillus Calmette-Guerin vaccination at birth and 2 months old age on the peripheral blood T-cell subpopulations [gamma/delta and alpha-beta T cell]. *Pediatr Allergy Immunol.* 2005;16:624–629.

69. Hoft DF, Brown RM, Roodman ST. Bacille Calmette-Guerin vaccination enhances human gamma delta T cell responsiveness to mycobacteria suggestive of a memory-like phenotype. *J Immunol.* 1998;161:1045–1054.

70. Kleinnijenhuis J, et al. BCG-induced trained immunity in NK cells: role for non-specific protection to infection. *Clin Immunol.* 2014;155:213–219.

71. Netea MG, et al. Trained immunity: a program of innate immune memory in health and disease. *Science.* 2016;352:aaf1098.

72. Quintin J, Cheng SC, van der Meer JW, Netea MG. Innate immune memory: towards a better understanding of host defense mechanisms. *Curr Opin Immunol.* 2014;29:1–7.

73. Quintin J, et al. Candida albicans infection affords protection against reinfection via functional reprogramming of monocytes. *Cell Host Microbe.* 2012;12:223–232.

74. Arts RJ, Joosten LA, Netea MG. Immunometabolic circuits in trained immunity. *Semin Immunol.* 2016;28(5):425–430.

75. Arts RJ, et al. Glutaminolysis and fumarate accumulation integrate immunometabolic and epigenetic programs in trained immunity. *Cell Metab.* 2016;24(6):807–819.

76. Cheng SC, et al. Broad defects in the energy metabolism of leukocytes underlie immunoparalysis in sepsis. *Nat Immunol.* 2016;17:406–413.

77. Novakovic B, et al. Beta-glucan reverses the epigenetic state of LPS-induced immunological tolerance. *Cell.* 2016;167:1354–1368.

78. Bekkering S, et al. Metabolic induction of trained immunity through the mevalonate pathway. *Cell.* 2018;172:135–146.

79. Lampropoulou V, et al. Itaconate links inhibition of succinate dehydrogenase with macrophage metabolic remodeling and regulation of inflammation. *Cell Metab.* 2016;24:158–166.

80. Lara-Astiaso D, et al. Immunogenetics. Chromatin state dynamics during blood formation. *Science.* 2014;345:943–949.

81. Saeed S, et al. Epigenetic programming of monocyte-to-macrophage differentiation and trained innate immunity. *Science.* 2014;345:1251086.

82. Ostuni R, et al. Latent enhancers activated by stimulation in differentiated cells. *Cell.* 2013;152:157–171.

83. Ghisletti S, et al. Identification and characterization of enhancers controlling the inflammatory gene expression program in macrophages. *Immunity.* 2010;32:317–328.

84. Cheng SC, et al. mTOR- and HIF-1alpha-mediated aerobic glycolysis as metabolic basis for trained immunity. *Science.* 2014;345:1250684.

85. Arts RJ, et al. Immunometabolic pathways in BCG-induced trained immunity. *Cell Rep.* 2016;17:2562–2571.

86. Kaufmann E, et al. BCG educates hematopoietic stem cells to generate protective innate immunity against tuberculosis. *Cell.* 2018;172:176–190. e119.

87. Crisan TO, et al. Uric acid priming in human monocytes is driven by the AKT-PRAS40 autophagy pathway. *Proc Natl Acad Sci USA.* 2017;114:5485–5490.

88. Flanagan KL, et al. Sex differences in the vaccine-specific and non-targeted effects of vaccines. *Vaccine.* 2011;29:2349–2354.

89. Schlums H, et al. Cytomegalovirus infection drives adaptive epigenetic diversification of NK cells with altered signaling and effector function. *Immunity.* 2015;42:443–456.

90. Verma D, et al. Anti-mycobacterial activity correlates with altered DNA methylation pattern in immune cells from BCG-vaccinated subjects. *Sci Rep.* 2017;7:12305.

CHAPTER 7

Nonspecific Effects of Neonatal Bacille Calmette-Guérin (BCG) Vaccination—From West African Observations to a Danish Randomized Clinical Trial

Thomas Nørrelykke Nissen*, Nina Marie Birk*, Jesper Kjærgaard[†]
*Department of Paediatrics, Copenhagen University Hospital, Hvidovre, Denmark
[†]The Department of Paediatrics and Adolescent Medicine, Juliane Marie Centret, Rigshospitalet, Copenhagen University Hospital, Copenhagen, Denmark

Contents

INTRODUCTION

The Bacille Calmette-Guérin (BCG) vaccine was introduced for use in humans in the 1920s after Albert Calmette and Camille Guérin succeeded in attenuating *Mycobacterium bovis*.[1] Today, the BCG vaccine is still the only licensed vaccine against tuberculosis (TB) and is used in routine vaccination programs in >100 countries.[2] The protection against TB is variable with lowest protection against adult pulmonary TB as opposed to disseminated TB and TB meningitis in childhood where evidence is well established.[3,4]

Shortly after the BCG vaccine was introduced in Sweden in the early 1920s, a regional physician named Carl Näslund made an unexpected observation.

The Value of BCG and TNF in Autoimmunity
https://doi.org/10.1016/B978-0-12-814603-3.00007-0

He noticed that the mortality of BCG-vaccinated children was significantly lower than the nonvaccinated children. As TB is, and was, a rare cause of death during childhood in Sweden, this was not expected to be caused by the protection against TB. It was concluded that the decreased mortality had to be due to protection against infections other than TB, and this was explained as "nonspecific immunity".[5]

Five decades later in the 1970s, it was discovered that BCG could be used in the treatment of bladder cancer, and BCG is now the primary adjuvant treatment of nonmuscle-invasive bladder cancer.[6] In the past few years, BCG has also been suggested for treatment of warts caused by Human Papilloma Virus,[7–9] cutaneous leishmaniasis,[10] multiple sclerosis,[11,12] and diabetes.[13]

During the past three decades, the initial observation made by Näslund has been investigated in West Africa. Clinical observational studies[14–17] and randomized clinical trials[18,19] showed that BCG vaccination decreased mortality at a magnitude that could not be explained by the protection against TB. Verbal autopsies showed that the effect was due to prevention of infections.[20] Other vaccines also seemed to have NSEs on mortality[21] and thus, the concept that vaccines can have health effects that extend beyond the protection against the target disease has now been coined NSEs of vaccines.[22] The idea of a nonspecific clinical effect after BCG vaccination is still controversial and breaks with the present understanding of how vaccines work.

The possibility that BCG and other vaccines could have NSEs on mortality, and therefore could impact the planning of vaccination programs, lead the WHO to commission a review of NSEs of vaccines in 2012.[23] On the basis of that report, the WHO working group concluded that BCG could have nonspecific effects, but more research should be conducted, preferably using a randomized trial design in other settings than the low-income, high burden of disease, high-mortality setting where most of the previous evidence was generated, and studies should look at a broader range of outcomes than mortality.[24]

The hypothesis of NSEs of BCG vaccination of neonates was then, for the first time, in a high-income setting with low prevalence of TB, investigated in a large-scale randomized clinical trial in Denmark. During 2012–15, 4262 children were randomized to neonatal BCG vaccination or control in The Danish Calmette Study to test whether BCG vaccination had NSEs on clinical outcomes and to study possible immunological mechanisms.[25]

THE SEARCH FOR AN IMMUNOLOGICAL EXPLANATION

Immunological Response to Neonatal BCG Vaccination

The local postvaccination reaction and possible adverse reactions following BCG vaccination are thoroughly described. Days to weeks after vaccination, an indurated papule appears at the site of vaccination. This may develop into a small pustule that, after weeks to months, heals with a small scar.[26] The immunological reaction to neonatal BCG vaccination on the other hand is less clear. It has been shown that BCG induces BCG-specific CD4 and CD8 T cells predominantly producing high levels of TH-1 cytokine IFN-γ,[27–29] as well as inducing low levels of TH-2 cytokines such as IL-4, IL-5, and IL-10.[30,31] In 10-week–old infants, it has been shown that BCG vaccination at birth also induces TNF-α, and the balance between induction of TH-1 cytokines as IFN-γ, TNF-α, and IL-2 and induction of TH-2 cytokines as IL-4 and IL-10 is dependent of route of administration[32] and strain.[33] In a randomized clinical trial from South Africa, it was shown that children BCG-vaccinated at 10 weeks old had a higher proportion of polyfunctional CD4 T cells coexpressing IFN-γ, TNF-α, and IL-2 when compared with children vaccinated at birth. This difference lasted for up to a year after vaccination, indicating that age of BCG vaccination also is a factor for the neonatal immune response to BCG vaccination.[34] Whereas the local reaction after BCG vaccination is well described, the immunological response and cytokine induction upon neonatal BCG vaccination is complex and still poorly understood, but immunologists suggest that heterologous immunity could be part of the explanation for nonspecific clinical effects.[35]

Heterologous Immunity

Heterologous immunity—defined as the phenomenon where previous exposure to a related or unrelated pathogen can alter the immune response to an infection—has been established over the past decades.[36] In vaccine trials, BCG has been investigated in the field of heterologous immunology as being the previous exposure. In both high- and low-income countries, BCG has been shown to alter the antibody response to subsequent vaccines, although results have been inconclusive.[27,37,38] A study in The Gambia showed that children who were BCG-vaccinated at birth had higher antibody response to hepatitis B vaccine at 4 months of age, where both BCG-vaccinated and control children had been hepatitis B-vaccinated at 0, 2, and 4 months of age.[27] An Australian study found an effect of BCG on pneumococcus conjugate vaccine (PCV) (serotype 9V and 18C) but a negative effect on hepatitis B antibodies.[37]

The effect of BCG on in vitro cytokine induction has been studied in several studies in West Africa.[27,39–41] In The Gambia, BCG vaccination at birth was associated with enhanced TH-1, TH-2, Tregs, IL-6, and IL-17 in mycobacterial cultures when compared with nonvaccinated children at age 4½ months.[41] Also in The Gambia, BCG enhanced IFN-γ, IL-5, and IL-13 production when stimulated in vitro with hepatitis B surface antigen (HBsAg) at 2 and 4½ months of age, when compared with control children.[27] In Guinea Bissau, a study found BCG to be associated with increased production of IL-1β, IL-6, TNF-α, and IFN-γ to innate stimulation with PMA and Pam3CSK4 when infants BCG-vaccinated at birth were compared with nonvaccinated controls at 4 weeks of age.[39]

Although several studies during the past decade have reported broader clinical effects of BCG than protection against TB, little focus has been on immunological mechanisms. Evidence of a more complex immune response and function is emerging, and research in both innate and adaptive mechanisms have led to possible explanations of nonspecific clinical effects of vaccines in general and BCG in particular.[42,43] Heterologous immunity has predominantly sought to explain T-cell cross-reactivity, but during the past 5 years, evidence of innate memory, termed "trained immunity", has also emerged as a possible explanation.[44]

T-Cell Cross-Reactivity

T-cell cross-reactivity is a well-known explanation for heterologous immunity within the classical paradigm of innate and adaptive immunity. In response to an encountered pathogen, an immune memory lymphocyte repertoire is created. This memory pool can generate an immune response to a subsequent pathogen if the antigens of the latter pathogen cross-reacts and stimulates the memory pool of the former encountered pathogen.[36] This has especially been studied in different virus infections, and one study showed that cross-reacting T cells are maintained in the memory pool after the subsequent unrelated infection, whereas noncross-reacting T cells are lost from the memory pool. This suggests that immune-dominance of memory T-cell epitopes are dependent of T-cell cross-reactivity with other nonrelated pathogens.[43,45]

Trained Immunity

New studies have shown that immune memory induced by heterologous immunological effects of BCG are also seen in innate cells of the immune system, which breaks with the paradigm of the immune system strictly divided into innate (no memory) and adaptive (memory) immunity. In 2012, Kleinnijenhuis et al. showed that heterologous immunity exists independently of the adaptive immune system. They showed that BCG-vaccinated mice depleted from T and B cells were protected from a lethal injection with *Candida albicans* when compared with nonvaccinated mice.[46] In adults, they also assessed the effect of BCG vaccination on cytokine response to in vitro stimulation with unrelated pathogens. They found that BCG vaccination induced monocyte-derived cytokines for up to 3 months, whereas heterologous effect of TH-1 and TH-17 cells lasted up to a year after vaccination.[47] These results indicated that phagocytic cells as monocytes, macrophages, and natural killer cells might play an important role in heterologous immunity.[48,49] In subsequent studies, the same group explored possible intracellular pathways and found that epigenetic reprogramming through changes in histone trimethylation at H3K4 induces changes in gene expression of the NOD2 receptor.[50] These changes led to alterations in both transcription of immune receptors and cytokine production,[51] thereby inducing memory to cells of the innate immune system as so-called "trained immunity".[50,52,53] In a recent small trial in neonates, it was found that the cytokine patter was different when assessing "trained immunity", indicating that neonates and adults develop different expressions of "trained immunity" after BCG vaccination.[54]

THE DANISH CALMETTE STUDY

To test the hypothesis of NSEs of neonatal BCG vaccination in a high-income setting, The Danish Calmette Study was initiated in 2012 and was conducted at three Danish University Hospitals; Rigshospitalet, Hvidovre Hospital, and Kolding Hospital. The main outcomes were all-cause hospitalization, parent-reported morbidity, and clinical findings with special focus on infections and atopic disease. Between October 2012 and November 2013, a total of 4262 newborn infants were included in the study. The study design was a randomized clinical trial with 1:1 allocation of newborn infants to BCG vaccination or no intervention. Inclusion criteria were gestational age (GA) >32 weeks, birth weight >1000 g, and written informed consent from both parents. Exclusion criteria were known immune deficiency, maternal intake of immune modulating medicine during pregnancy, severe illness of the child, major malformation in the child, and no Danish-speaking parent.

During the second or third trimester, a letter with information about the study was sent to mothers planning to give birth at one of the three study sites. Subsequently, the mothers were contacted by telephone by the study staff to give verbal information and answer questions about the study. If the families gave verbal consent for study participation, a background interview was made and they were instructed to return a signed consent form.

Within 7 days of birth, infants were randomized to BCG-vaccination or no intervention. If randomized to vaccination, the BCG vaccine was applied intradermally on the upper lateral part of the left shoulder. The BCG vaccine was applied in a standard dose of 0.05 mL as recommended for children, and BCG SSI strain 1331 was used as intervention in all children.

At 3 months of age, the families were interviewed by telephone to answer questions about episodes of illness, growth, medication, and routine vaccinations. Subsequently, children were invited to the study facility for a clinical examination with focus on eczema, wheeze, and assessment of anthropometrics. At 13 months of age, the families were again contacted by telephone to answer questions about episodes of illness, medication, use of health care services, growth and development, and routine vaccinations. Subsequently the children were again invited to the study facility for a clinical examination. At both clinical examinations, the families of both vaccinated and control infants were instructed to cover the site of vaccination. At the end of the final clinical examination, the vaccination site was revealed and the scar size was measured.[55]

Clinical Findings
Hospitalization and Infectious Diseases
Previously, the most compelling evidence of NSEs of BCG vaccination in children had been on mortality following severe infections in the low-income setting of Guinea-Bissau.[17,18,56] To study whether BCG vaccination at birth had effects on child health in a high-income setting, it was necessary to study morbidity instead of mortality, because the under-5-years-old mortality rate in Denmark is 3.5 of 1000 and 123.9 of 1000 in Guinea-Bissau.[57]

The previous trials from West Africa had used all-cause mortality as an outcome, and for the Danish Calmette Study, all-cause hospitalization up to age 15 months was chosen as the main outcome, supplemented by specific infectious morbidity outcomes, such as hospitalization for infectious diseases (Stensballe et al., manuscript under review JPIDS) and parent-reported infections,[58] as well as eczema and wheeze.[59,60]

The trial did not show any effect of BCG vaccination at birth on all-cause hospitalizations[61] or on hospitalizations for infectious diseases (Stensballe et al., in review JPIDS) in the prespecified follow-up period at age 15 months. Neither was there an overall effect on parent-reported infections. In a subgroup analysis of children of mothers who had been previously vaccinated with BCG, there was an incidence rate ratio of 0.62 (0.39–0.98) for infections from 0 to 3 months, corresponding to a number needed to vaccinate of 14,[58] and for infectious disease hospitalization an incidence rate ratio of 0.65 (0.45–0.94) (Stensballe et al., in review JPIDS), thus indicating that maternal priming with BCG could be a prerequisite for the nonspecific effect of BCG. This hypothesis is currently being explored in Guinea-Bissau. An observational study from Greenland, where BCG vaccination has been in use since 1955, utilized a transient halt in BCG vaccination from 1991 to 1996 to compare hospitalization rates between BCG-vaccinated and BCG-unvaccinated children from 3 months to 3 years in a population where most of the mothers would have been BCG-vaccinated themselves. This study did not find an effect of BCG vaccination on hospitalization,[62] but in the Danish Calmette Study, the possible effect was most pronounced under age 3 months and also seemed to be very early in a randomized trial from Guinea-Bissau.[18]

Atopy and Allergic Diseases

Besides NSEs on mortality and morbidity in children, BCG vaccination has been associated with decreased risk of atopic diseases.[63,64] For this reason, the Danish Calmette Study also studied atopy as a secondary outcome. In the Danish Calmette Study, randomization to neonatal BCG vaccination marginally reduced the incidence of atopic dermatitis by age 13 months (RR = 0.90 (0.80–1.00)). In the subgroup of children with atopic predisposition, neonatal BCG reduced the incidence of atopic dermatitis with number needed to treat of 21 (CI: 12–71). We found a tendency for a beneficial effect of BCG on atopic dermatitis in the 17% of BCG-vaccinated mothers, the effect estimate = 0.77 (0.58–1.01), thus also indicating that perhaps maternal priming may play a role.[60] There was no effect of BCG vaccination on the incidence of recurrent wheeze, allergic sensitization, or suspected food allergy at age 13 months, either in the total population or in the subgroup of children where the mother was BCG-vaccinated herself.[59,65]

Adverse Reactions and Scar Development

The normal reaction following BCG vaccination is thoroughly described, as well as the possible adverse reactions after BCG vaccination. Because the study set-up was investigation of BCG vaccination for purposes other than prevention of TB, adverse reactions had to be monitored and reported to local health authorities. This also gave us the opportunity to assess adverse reactions to neonatal BCG vaccination in a high-income setting with low prevalence of TB and HIV, and where BCG vaccination is not part of the routine vaccination program.[66]

When children were examined at 13 months of age, 91% of the BCG-vaccinated children had developed a scar at the site of vaccination, and no child experienced disseminated BCG disease during the follow-up period. Of the 2118 BCG-vaccinated children, suppurative lymphadenitis was registered in 10 children. All children presented with lymphadenitis in the axilla as their primary symptom, and the onset of symptoms ranged from 25 to 200 days after BCG vaccination. All cases healed with a scar, but the time from onset of symptoms to development of a scar ranged from 63 to 328 days. The rate of suppurative lymphadenitis was five times higher than expected from the summary of product characteristics, but all children were successfully treated conservatively without use of antibiotics or surgical intervention.

When parents at the end of the study were asked if they agreed with the statement: "We are satisfied with our decision of having our child BCG vaccinated", 94% of the parents to BCG-vaccinated children not experiencing suppurative or regional lymphadenitis agreed or strongly agreed. Among parents to children experiencing suppurative lymphadenitis, only 70% agreed or strongly agreed.

Immunological Findings

Thymus Size

The thymus is essential in developing a normal functioning immune system as the maturation of T cells takes place within the thymic microenvironment.[67] In Guinea-Bissau, the size of the thymus, measured as the thymic index (TI), has been linked to infant survival. In 6-month-old infants, a doubling of TI was associated with a 72% reduction in mortality up to the age of 36 months.[68] To test if thymic size was affected by BCG vaccination, and thereby potentially represent a immunological link between BCG and reduced mortality, thymic size was examined in a subgroup of infants within The Danish Calmette Study. By transsternal ultrasound,[69] the absolute volume index (TI) and the relative volume index, thymic weight index (TWI), were assessed. A total of 314 infants were scanned at baseline before vaccination of the intervention group, but after randomization, 301 infants were scanned at the 3 months follow-up. No difference in either TI or TWI was found at age 3 months between the BCG and the control group; the geometric mean ratio (GMR) was 0.96, 95% CI (0.89–1.02) for TI and 0.96, 95% CI (0.90–1.02) for TWI. Adjusting for infant weight at baseline, baseline characteristics did not change the estimates. None of the prespecified effect modifiers, including sex, scar (yes/no), maternal BCG, and time of vaccination, influenced the statistical nonsignificant relation between thymic size and BCG.[70]

T- and B-Cell Subpopulations

To examine the effect of BCG on essential T-cell functions, we assessed alterations in flow cytometry-determined phenotypes of T and B cells in peripheral blood. The phenotypes were divided into groups according to effector function: *immune regulation* (regulatory T cells (Tregs), Th17 cells, Tc17 cells, and CD19+CD24highCD38high B cells), *naïve cells and thymic output* (naïve cells and recent thymic emigrants (RTE)), and *T-cell homeostasis* (central memory cells, effector memory cells, late differentiated cells, chronic activated cells, and apoptotic cells). Blood samples were taken 4 ($\pm$2) days after randomization and at 3 and 13 months of age. A total of 114 infants were examined 4 ($\pm$2) days postrandomization, and 106 infants were examined at 3 and 13 months of age. We found no overall effects on either naïve cells and cells reflecting thymic output or in immune regulatory cells. In cells in the category of T-cell homeostasis, an effect was found in effector memory T cells (TEM), late differentiated T cells (LDC), and apoptotic T cells. At 3 months, the proportion of TEM was higher in the BCG group compared with the control group for both CD4+ T cells (GMR 1.62, 95% CI (1.20–2.21), $P=0.002$) and CD8+ T cells (GMR 1.69, 95% CI (1.06–2.70), $P=0.03$). The same effects was seen for absolute counts of CD4+ cells (GMR 1.64, 95% CI (1.21–2.23), $P=0.002$). At 13 months of age, fewer LDC CD4+ T cells were seen in BCG-vaccinated infants than in controls for both proportions (GMR 0.62, 95% CI (0.38–1.00), $P=0.05$) and absolute cell counts (GMR 0.59, 95% CI (0.38–0.93), $P=0.02$). Furthermore, a decrease was found in both proportions of apoptotic CD4+ T cells (GMR 0.55, 95% CI (0.32–0.92), $P=0.03$) and absolute counts (GMR 0.53, 95% CI (0.31–0.91), $P=0.02$) in BCG-vaccinated infants compared with controls.[71]

   B cells with the phenotype CD19+CD24highCD38high are often referred to as B-regulatory cells and have been shown to be enriched for IL-10.[72] In an analysis of effect modification, the effect of BCG differed by sex in CD19+CD24highCD38high B cells at 13 months; GMR for boys was 0.89, 95% CI (0.75–1.05), and for girls, GMR 1.26, 95% CI (1.06–1.50), P value for interaction = 0.005.

When looking at effect modification by time of randomization, as either early (0–1 days) or late (2–7 days), BCG increased proportions of Tregs at all three time points following early vaccination, with the opposite effect following late vaccination.

Overall, we found limited impact of neonatal BCG vaccination on lymphocyte subsets. The increase in effector memory cells at 3 months indicates antigen encounter and may be associated to development of specific memory representing the specific effect of the vaccine. The time differential effect found in Tregs may be assessed in future studies, with potential significance in both the fields of autoimmune disease[73] and vaccine immunogenicity in early life.[74]

Antibody Response to Subsequent Vaccines

To investigate the hypothesis that BCG vaccination influences the antibody response to subsequently given vaccines, 300 children were included in an analysis of specific antibody responses. All children received PCV, Prevenar 13, and penta valent or hexa valent vaccines (DiTeKiPol/Act-Hib or Infanrixhexa) at 3, 5, and 12 months of age. Children were bled at 13 months of age, and specific vaccine antibodies were measured in serum using Luminex xMAP technology.[38]

For all measured antibodies, 96%–100% of the children had antibody levels above the protection limit, and BCG vaccination was not associated with having a specific IgG above the protection limit. Overall, no effect of BCG vaccination was seen on antibody levels after vaccination with DiTeKiPol/Act-Hib or Infanrixhexa with a GMR of antipertussis toxin (PT) IgG 1.11 (95% CI 0.91–1.36), antidiphtheria toxoid (DT) IgG 0.97 (95% CI 0.81–1.16), antitetanus toxin (TT) IgG 0.92 (95% CI 0.76–1.12), and antihaemophilus influenza type b (Hib) IgG 0.84 (95% CI 0.58–1.21). Also no effect of BCG vaccination was seen on antibody levels after PCV vaccination, although IgG tended to be higher for serotype 6b, 14, 18c, and 23f in the BCG group, whereas serotype 4, 9v, and 19f tended to be lower.

When analyzing the data with "age of randomization" as an effect modifier of BCG vaccination, BCG was associated with higher IgG levels in children randomized on day 2–7, whereas the opposite was seen in children randomized on day 0–1. For anti-PT IgG, the effect of BCG vaccination on GMR was 0.91 (95% CI 0.70–1.18) at day 0–1 and 1.47 (95% CI 1.08–2.00) at day 2–7 (P-value = 0.02 for interaction between "age at randomization" groups). For anti-Hib IgG, the group randomized on day 0–1 had a GMR of 0.64 (95% CI 0.40–1.05) compared with a GMR of 1.2 (95% CI 0.68–2.12) in the group randomized on day 2–7 (P-value = 0.1 for interaction between "age at randomization" groups). In the analysis of specific antibodies against PCV, the effect modification was statistically significant for three serotypes: serotype 9v, with a GMR of 0.76 (95% CI 0.58–1.00) at day 0–1 and 1.38 (95% CI 1.00–1.91) at day 2–7 (P-value = 0.005 for interaction between "age at randomization" groups); serotype 18c, with a GMR of 0.92 (95% CI 0.70–1.21) at day 0–1 and 1.55 (95% CI 1.12–2.13) at day 2–7 (P-value = 0.02 for interaction between "age at randomization" groups); and serotype 19f, with a GMR of 0.78 (95% CI 0.59–1.03) at day 0–1 and 1.41 (95% CI 1.02–1.96) at day 2–7 (P-value = 0.007 for interaction between "age at randomization" groups).

In the overall analysis, we found no effect of neonatal BCG vaccination on antibody response to subsequent vaccines during the first year of life. However, interaction analysis indicates that an effect is present if neonates are BCG vaccinated later than the first 2 days of life.

Cytokine Production

In a substudy, 158 children (80 BCG; 78 controls) were bled for the purpose of investigating cytokine response to BCG nonrelated pathogens. They were bled 4 days after randomization (short-term effect), 3 months old just before introduction of other childhood vaccines (long-term effect of BCG), and 13 months old after completion of DiTeKiPol/Act-Hib and Prevenar 13 vaccination at 3, 5, and 12 months (long-term effect). At each time point, whole blood was cultured with RPMI (neg), lipopolysaccharide (LPS), phytohaemagglutinin (PHA), *Escherichia coli*, *Streptococcus pneumoniae*, *C. albicans*, and BCG. Cytokines were measured in supernatants of whole blood stimulated for 24 h (TNF-α, IL-1β, and IL-6) or 96 h (IFN-γ, IL-17, IL-22, and IL-10). Cytokine levels were measured using commercially available enzyme-linked immunosorbent assay (ELISA) kits.[75]

Overall, we found no effect of neonatal BCG vaccination on cytokine production after whole blood stimulation. At 13 months, we did find an effect of BCG, which resulted in low levels of IL-1β (GMR 0.54, CI: 0.32–0.92, P = 0.02), higher levels of IL-22 (GMR 3.70, CI: 2.49–5.48, $P < 0.001$), and higher levels of IFN-γ. GMR was 7.98 (95% CI 5.80–10.98, P-value <0.001). Although we found an expected effect of BCG vaccination on IFN-γ response to BCG stimulation, the magnitude of the response was much lower than expected. The geometric mean concentration (GMC) in the BCG group was 144 pg/mL, and when creating a cut-off where 95%

of the control children responded below, only 54% of the BCG-vaccinated children had a higher response.

To test "age at randomization" as an effect modifier of BCG vaccination, the children were divided into two groups: randomized on day 0–1 or randomized on day 2–7. In the 4-day samples, IL-1β, TNF-α, IL-6, IL-10, and IL-22 were higher in the BCG group compared with controls among infants randomized on day 2–7, whereas the opposite was seen in the group randomized on day 0–1. This tendency was statistically significant for TNF-α to *E. coli* and LPS stimulation ($P = 0.05$ and 0.03), IL-6 to *E. coli*, PHA and LPS stimulation ($P = 0.001, 0.003$, and 0.001), and IL-10 to S. pneumoniae PHA and LPS stimulation ($P = 0.04, 0.04$, and 0.03). In the 3- and 13-month samples, this tendency of effect modification was not seen.

We were not able to confirm a BCG-induced change in the cytokine production after stimulation with BCG nonrelated antigens and pathogens. However, in the 4-day samples, we saw an opposite effect of BCG vaccination in favor of being vaccinated on day 2–7 compared with children vaccinated on day 0–1.

DISCUSSION

The lack of effect on prevention of infections in the Danish Calmette Study was unexpected in the light of the previous research on nonspecific prevention of infections.[76–80] There are several possible explanations for this finding. One could be that the immune response to BCG differs according to geographical location and setting,[81] as well as exposure to other mycobacteria,[82] both of which differs significantly between the high-income setting of the Danish Calmette Study and where most of the previous research has been done. Also the pathogens and severity of infections are different between high- and low-income settings. There was indication of NSEs, particularly in the subgroup of children where the mother was BCG-vaccinated herself, and another possible explanation for the differing results could also be that most of the previous research has been conducted in settings[21,23] where maternal exposure to BCG or environmental mycobacteria is more frequent, or in high-income settings where BCG vaccination is part of the public vaccination program.[83] An exception is a study from Greenland where maternal priming was present, which did not show a nonspecific effect on hospitalization among the children, even though this study did not look at the first 3 months, where the children had not received any other vaccinations and where NSEs of BCG seem to be most pronounced.[84] In terms of prevention of TB, no particular BCG strain is deemed superior to the others, although the strains differ in both immune response and adverse reactions.[85] Using BCG SSI strain 1331 in a Danish population revealed a higher incidence of suppurative lymphadenitis. However, little is known about the correlation of adverse reactions and nonspecific clinical effects, scar development, and nonspecific immunological effects, but a recent study from Guinea-Bissau found that, also within the BCG SSI strain 1331, they found differences in scar formation and cytokine responses between batches of the same strain.[86]

A review by the Strategic Advisory Group of Experts (SAGE) on immunization on nonspecific prevention of morbidity and mortality after BCG vaccination concluded that the present evidence suggests a clinical important NSE of neonatal BCG vaccination.[23] The SAGE review of studies with immunological outcomes were only able to conclude that some studies showed consistent direction of IFN-γ response and lymphoproliferation to microbial antigen stimulation suggestive of a nonspecific immunological effect. However, the studies included in the review differed too much in study design to allow a meta-analysis of the data.[87] Within the immunological studies in The Danish Calmette Study, no consistent nonspecific immunological effects of neonatal BCG vaccination were found. In preplanned secondary analysis, we did however find some consistent indicators. In most clinical trials on BCG vaccination, the chosen time point for vaccination is at the time of birth. Our results across the analysis of vaccine,specific antibody response, cytokine response, and effects on T- and B-cell subsets in The Danish Calmette Study indicate that the nonspecific effect of neonatal BCG vaccination may differ depending on time of vaccination within days after birth.[38,71,75]

The relationship between immune characteristics of the BCG vaccine and specific and nonspecific clinical effects, as well as the broad range of immunological markers such as IFN-γ response, induction of trained immunity, scar development, and tuberculin skin test reaction, still needs to be explored. In The Danish Calmette Study, we found a high frequency of adverse reactions and scar development but poor effect of inducing IFN-γ response to in vitro BCG stimulation. This highlights the need for a standardized approach of how we assess and interpret the relationship between different clinical and immunological outcomes in BCG vaccine trials.

Future studies on biological material collected during the first year of life from children in The Danish Calmette Study who participated in the immunological studies are planned. In collaboration with the Human

Functional Genomics Project,[88] microbiome, proteomics, genetics, and functional analysis of epigenetic changes will be investigated. This will provide novel information not only on the effect of BCG but also the development of the immune system during the first year of life.

CONCLUSIONS

The Danish Calmette Study is the first large, high-quality randomized trial to be conducted in a high-income setting evaluating the NSEs of BCG. The trial did not provide evidence of a public health benefit concerning prevention of infections or atopic diseases in a high-income setting, nor did it find nonspecific immunological effects, as opposed to consistent findings in low-income settings. When setting up trials to study both clinical and immunological NSEs, future studies should take into consideration maternal BCG vaccination, age of vaccination, BCG strain, environmental mycobacteria, and the possible implication of other routine vaccines given throughout childhood.

REFERENCES

1. Locht C. The history of BCG. In: Nor NM, Acosta A, Sarmiento ME, eds. *The Art & Science of Tuberculosis Vaccine Development*. 1st ed. Selangor Darul Ehsan: Oxford University Press; 2010.
2. Ottenhoff THM, Kaufmann SHE. Vaccines against tuberculosis: where are we and where do we need to go? *PLoS Pathog*. 2012;8(5),e1002607.
3. Roy A, Eisenhut M, Harris RJ, Rodrigues LC. Effect of BCG vaccination against *Mycobacterium tuberculosis* infection in children: systematic review and meta-analysis. *Open Access*. 2014;4643(August):1–11.
4. Trunz BB, Fine P, Dye C. Effect of BCG vaccination on childhood tuberculous meningitis and miliary tuberculosis worldwide: a meta-analysis and assessment of cost-effectiveness. *Lancet*. 2006;367(9517):1173–1180.
5. Naeslund C. Expérience de vaccination par le bcg dans la province du norrbotten (suède). *Rev Tuberc*. 1931;12:617–636.
6. Askeland EJ, Newton MR, O'Donnell MA, Luo Y. Bladder cancer immunotherapy: BCG and beyond. *Adv Urol*. 2012;2012:181987.
7. Salem A, Nofal A, Hosny D. Treatment of common and plane warts in children with topical viable Bacillus Calmette-Guerin. *Pediatr Dermatol*. 2013;30(1):60–63.
8. Nofal A, Yosef A, Salah E. Treatment of recalcitrant warts with Bacillus Calmette-Guérin: a promising new approach. *Dermatol Ther*. 2013;26(6):481–485.
9. Metawea B, El-Nashar A-R, Kamel I, Kassem W, Shamloul R. Application of viable bacille Calmette-Guérin topically as a potential therapeutic modality in condylomata acuminata: a placebo-controlled study. *Urology*. 2005;65(2):247–250.
10. Pereira LIA, Dorta ML, Pereira AJCS, et al. Increase of NK cells and proinflammatory monocytes are associated with the clinical improvement of diffuse cutaneous leishmaniasis after immunochemotherapy with BCG/Leishmania antigens. *Am J Trop Med Hyg*. 2009;81(3):378–383.

11. Paolillo A, Buzzi MG, Giugni E, et al. The effect of Bacille Calmette-Guérin on the evolution of new enhancing lesions to hypointense T1 lesions in relapsing remitting MS. *J Neurol*. 2003;250(2):247–248.

12. Ristori G, Romano S, Cannoni S, et al. Effects of Bacille Calmette-Guérin after the first demyelinating event in the CNS. *Neurology*. 2014;82(1):41–48.

13. Faustman DL, Wang L, Okubo Y, et al. Proof-of-concept, randomized, controlled clinical trial of Bacillus Calmette-Guerin for treatment of long-term type 1 diabetes. *PLoS One*. 2012;7(8), e41756.

14. Roth A, Gustafson P, Nhaga A, et al. BCG vaccination scar associated with better childhood survival in Guinea-Bissau. *Int J Epidemiol*. 2005;34(3):540–547.

15. Roth A, Sodemann M, Jensen H, et al. Tuberculin reaction, BCG scar, and lower female mortality. *Epidemiology*. 2006;17(5):562–568.

16. Storgaard L, Rodrigues A, Martins C, et al. Development of BCG scar and subsequent morbidity and mortality in rural Guinea-Bissau. *Clin Infect Dis*. 2015;61(6):950–959.

17. Kristensen I, Aaby P, Jensen H. Routine vaccinations and child survival: follow up study in Guinea-Bissau, West Africa. *BMJ*. 2000;321(7274):1435–1438.

18. Aaby P, Roth A, Ravn H, et al. Randomized trial of BCG vaccination at birth to low-birth-weight children: beneficial nonspecific effects in the neonatal period? *J Infect Dis*. 2011;204(2):245–252.

19. Biering-Sørensen S, Aaby P, Lund N, et al. Early BCG-Denmark and neonatal mortality among infants weighing <2500 g: a randomized controlled trial. *Clin Infect Dis*. 2017;65(7):1183–1190.

20. Flanagan KL, van Crevel R, Curtis N, Shann F, Levy O. Heterologous ("nonspecific") and sex-differential effects of vaccines: epidemiology, clinical trials, and emerging immunologic mechanisms. *Clin Infect Dis*. 2013;1–7.

21. Shann F. The non-specific effects of vaccines. *Arch Dis Child*. 2010;95(9):662–667.

22. Aaby P, Benn CS. Non-specific and sex-differential effects of routine vaccines: what evidence is needed to take these effects into consideration in low-income countries? *Hum Vaccin*. 2011;7(1):120–124.

23. Higgins J, Soares-Weiser K, Reingold A. Systematic review of the non-specific effects of BCG, DTP and measles containing vaccines. *Wkly Epidemiol Rec*. 2014;89(May):1–34.

24. Evidence based recommendations on non-specific effects of BCG, DTP-containing and measles-containing vaccines on mortality in children under 5 years of age. In: SAGE Non-Specific Effects of Vaccine Working Group; 2014.

25. Thøstesen LM, Nissen TN, Kjærgaard J, et al. Bacillus Calmette-Guérin immunisation at birth and morbidity among Danish children: a prospective, randomised, clinical trial. *Contemp Clin Trials*. 2015;42:213–218.

26. SSI. *BCG Vaccine "SSI"*. Available from http://www.produktresume.dk/docushare/dsweb/GetRendition/Document-13163/html; 2015.

27. Ota MOC, Vekemans J, Schlegel-Haueter SE, et al. Influence of *Mycobacterium bovis* Bacillus Calmette-Guerin on antibody and cytokine responses to human neonatal vaccination. *J Immunol*. 2002;168(2):919–925.

28. Marchant A, Goetghebuer T, Ota MO, et al. Newborns develop a Th1-type immune response to *Mycobacterium bovis* Bacillus Calmette-Guerin vaccination. *J Immunol*. 1999;163(4):2249–2255.

29. Murray RA, Mansoor N, Harbacheuski R, et al. Bacillus Calmette-Guerin vaccination of human newborns induces a specific, functional CD8+ T cell response. *J Immunol*. 2006;177(8):5647–5651.

30. Power CA, Wei G, Bretscher PA. Mycobacterial dose defines the Th1/Th2 nature of the immune response independently of whether immunization is administered by the intravenous, subcutaneous, or intradermal route. *Infect Immun*. 1998;66(12):5743–5750.

31. Hussey GD, Watkins MLV, Goddard EA, et al. Neonatal mycobacterial specific cytotoxic T-lymphocyte and cytokine profiles in response to distinct BCG vaccination strategies. *Immunology*. 2002;105(3):314–324.

32. Davids V, Hanekom WA, Mansoor N, et al. The effect of Bacille Calmette-Guérin vaccine strain and route of administration on induced immune responses in vaccinated infants. *J Infect Dis*. 2006;193(4):531–536.

33. Ritz N, Dutta B, Donath S, et al. The influence of Bacille Calmette-Guérin vaccine strain on the immune response against tuberculosis. *Am J Respir Crit Care Med*. 2012;185(2):213–222. https://doi.org/10.1164/rccm.201104-0714OC.

34. Kagina BMN, Abel B, Bowmaker M, et al. Delaying BCG vaccination from birth to 10 weeks of age may result in an enhanced memory CD4 T cell response. *Vaccine*. 2009;27:5488–5495.

35. Soares AP, Scriba TJ, Joseph S, et al. Bacille Calmette Guerin vaccination of human newborns induces T cells with complex cytokine and phenotypic profiles. *J Immunol*. 2008;180(5):3569–3577.

36. Welsh RM, Selin LK. No one is naive: the significance of heterologous T-cell immunity. *Nat Rev Immunol*. 2002;2(6):417–426.

37. Ritz N, Mui M, Balloch A, Curtis N. Non-specific effect of Bacille Calmette-Guérin vaccine on the immune response to routine immunisations. *Vaccine*. 2013;2885–2889.

38. Nissen TN, Birk NM, Smits G, et al. Bacille Calmette-Guérin (BCG) vaccination at birth and antibody responses to childhood vaccines. A randomised clinical trial. *Vaccine*. 2017;35:2084–2091.

39. Jensen KJ, Larsen N, Biering-Sørensen S, et al. Heterologous immunological effects of early BCG vaccination in low-birth-weight infants in Guinea-Bissau: a randomized-controlled trial. *J Infect Dis*. 2015;211(6):956–967.

40. Vekemans J, Amedei A, Ota MO, et al. Neonatal Bacillus Calmette-Guérin vaccination induces adult-like IFN-gamma production by CD4+ T lymphocytes. *Eur J Immunol*. 2001;31(5):1531–1535.

41. Burl S, Adetifa UJ, Cox M, et al. Delaying bacillus Calmette-Guérin vaccination from birth to 4 1/2 months of age reduces postvaccination Th1 and IL-17 responses but leads to comparable mycobacterial responses at 9 months of age. *J Immunol*. 2010;185(4):2620–2628.

42. Benn CS, Netea MG, Selin LK, Aaby P. A small jab—a big effect: nonspecific immunomodulation by vaccines. *Trends Immunol*. 2013;34(9):431–439.

43. Gil A, Kenney LL, Mishra R, Watkin LB, Aslan N, Selin LK. Vaccination and heterologous immunity: educating the immune system. *Trans R Soc Trop Med Hyg*. 2014;109(1):62–69.

44. Netea MG, Joosten LAB, Latz E, et al. Trained immunity: a program of innate immune memory in health and disease. *Science*. 2016;352(6284), aaf1098. https://doi.org/10.1126/science.aaf1098.

45. M a B, Pinto AK, K a D, Schneck JP, Welsh RM, Selin LK. T cell immunodominance and maintenance of memory regulated by unexpectedly cross-reactive pathogens. *Nat Immunol*. 2002;3(7):627–634.

46. Kleinnijenhuis J, Quintin J, Preijers F, et al. Bacille Calmette-Guerin induces NOD2-dependent nonspecific protection from reinfection via epigenetic reprogramming of monocytes. *Proc Natl Acad Sci U S A*. 2012;109(43):17537–17542.

47. Kleinnijenhuis J, Quintin J, Preijers F, Benn CS, Joosten L. a B, Jacobs C, et al. Long-lasting effects of BCG vaccination on both heterologous Th1/Th17 responses and innate trained immunity. *J Innate Immun*. 2014;6(2):152–158.

48. Buffen K, Oosting M, Quintin J, et al. Autophagy controls BCG-induced trained immunity and the response to intravesical BCG therapy for bladder cancer. *PLoS Pathog*. 2014;10(10).

49. Kleinnijenhuis J, Quintin J, Preijers F, Joosten L. a B, Jacobs C, Xavier RJ, et al. BCG-induced trained immunity in NK cells: role for non-specific protection to infection. *Clin Immunol*. 2014;155(2):213–219.

50. Quintin J, Cheng S-C, van der Meer JW, Netea MG. Innate immune memory: towards a better understanding of host defense mechanisms. *Curr Opin Immunol.* 2014;29C:1–7.
51. Kleinnijenhuis J, van Crevel R, Netea MG. Trained immunity: consequences for the heterologous effects of BCG vaccination. *Trans R Soc Trop Med Hyg.* 2015;109(1):29–35. https://doi.org/10.1093/trstmh/tru168.
52. Netea MG, Quintin J, van der Meer JW. Trained immunity: a memory for innate host defense. *Cell Host Microbe.* 2011;9(5):355–361. https://doi.org/10.1016/j.chom.2011.04.006.
53. Blok BA, Arts RJW, van Crevel R, Benn CS, Netea MG. Trained innate immunity as underlying mechanism for the long-term, nonspecific effects of vaccines. *J Leukoc Biol.* 2015;98(3):347–356.
54. Smith SG, Kleinnijenhuis J, Netea MG, Dockrell HM. Whole Blood Profiling of Bacillus Calmette-Guérin-induced trained innate immunity in infants identifies epidermal growth factor, IL-6, platelet-derived growth factor-AB/BB, and natural killer cell activation. *Front Immunol.* 2017;8(June):1–11.
55. Thøstesen LM, Nissen TN, Kjærgaard J, et al. Bacillus Calmette-Guérin immunisation at birth and morbidity among Danish children: a prospective, randomised, clinical trial. *Contemp Clin Trials.* 2015;42:213–218.
56. Higgins J, Soares-Weiser K, Reingold A. *Systematic Review of the Non-Specific Effects of BCG, DTP and Measles Containing Vaccines*; 2014.1–34.
57. 2015 Child Mortality Collaborators GBD. Global, regional, national, and selected subnational levels of stillbirths, neonatal, infant, and under-5 mortality, 1980–2015: a systematic analysis for the Global Burden of Disease Study 2015. *Lancet (Lond, Engl).* 2016;388(10053):1725–1774.
58. Kjærgaard J, Birk NM, Nissen TN, et al. Nonspecific effect of BCG vaccination at birth on early childhood infections: a randomized, clinical multicenter trial. *Pediatr Res.* 2016;80(August):1–5.
59. Thøstesen LM, Stensballe LG, Pihl GT, et al. Neonatal BCG-vaccination has no effect on recurrent wheeze in the first year of life. A randomized clinical trial. *J Allergy Clin Immunol.* 2017;(2017).
60. Thøstesen LM, Kjaergaard J, Pihl GT, et al. Neonatal BCG-vaccination and atopic dermatitis before 13 months of age. A randomised clinical trial. *Allergy.* 2017;38(1):42–49. https://doi.org/10.1111/ijlh.12426.
61. Stensballe LG, Sørup S, Aaby P, et al. BCG vaccination at birth and early childhood hospitalisation: a randomised clinical multicentre trial. *Arch Dis Child.* 2016;archdischild-2016-310760. https://doi.org/10.1136/archdischild-2016-310760.
62. Haahr S, Michelsen SW, Andersson M, et al. Non-specific effects of BCG vaccination on morbidity among children in Greenland: a population-based cohort study. *Int J Epidemiol.* 2016;dyw244. https://doi.org/10.1093/ije/dyw244.
63. Arnoldussen DL, Linehan M, Sheikh A. BCG vaccination and allergy: a systematic review and meta-analysis. *J Allergy Clin Immunol.* 2011;127(1):246–253. 253-21.
64. Linehan MF, Nurmatov U, Frank TL, Niven RM, Baxter DN, Sheikh A. Does BCG vaccination protect against childhood asthma? Final results from the Manchester Community Asthma Study retrospective cohort study and updated systematic review and meta-analysis. *J Allergy Clin Immunol.* 2014;133(3).688–95.e14. https://doi.org/10.1016/j.jaci.2013.08.007.
65. Thøstesen LM, Kjaer HF, Pihl GT, et al. Neonatal BCG has no effect on allergic sensitization and suspected food allergy until 13 months. *Pediatr Allergy Immunol.* 2017;38(1):42–49.
66. Nissen TN, Birk NM, Kjærgaard J, et al. Adverse reactions to the Bacillus Calmette-Guérin (BCG) vaccine in new-born infants—an evaluation of the Danish strain 1331 SSI in a randomized clinical trial. *Vaccine.* 2016;34(22):2477–2482.
67. Savino W. The thymus is a common target organ in infectious diseases. *PLoS Pathog.* 2006;2(6):0472–0483.

68. Garly ML, Trautner SL, Marx C, et al. Thymus size at 6 months of age and subsequent child mortality. *J Pediatr*. 2008;153(5).
69. Hasselbalch H, Nielsen MB, Jeppesen D, Pedersen JF, Karkov J. Sonographic measurement of the thymus in infants. *Eur Radiol*. 1996;6(5):700–703.
70. Birk NM, Nissen TN, Zingmark V, et al. Bacillus Calmette-Guérin vaccination, thymic size and thymic output in healthy newborns. *Pediatr Res*. 2017;.
71. Birk NM, Nissen TN, Kjærgaard J, et al. Effects of Bacillus Calmette-Guérin (BCG) vaccination at birth on T and B lymphocyte subsets: results from a clinical randomized trial. *Sci Rep*. 2017;7(1):12398.
72. Blair P, Noreña LY, Flores-Borja F, et al. CD19+CD24hiCD38hi B cells exhibit regulatory capacity in healthy individuals but are functionally impaired in systemic lupus erythematosus patients. *Immunity*. 2010;32:129–140.
73. Noack M, Miossec P. Th17 and regulatory T cell balance in autoimmune and inflammatory diseases. *Autoimmun Rev*. 2014;13(6):668–677.
74. Ndure J, Flanagan KL. Targeting regulatory T cells to improve vaccine immunogenicity in early life. *Front Microbiol*. 2014;5(September):477.
75. Nissen TN, Birk NM, Blok BA, et al. Bacillus Calmette-Guérin vaccination at birth and in vitro cytokine responses to non-specific stimulation. A randomized clinical trial. *Eur J Clin Microbiol Infect Dis*. 2018;37(1):29–41.
76. Roth A, Gustafson P, Nhaga A, et al. BCG vaccination scar associated with better childhood survival in Guinea-Bissau. *Int J Epidemiol*. 2005;34(3):540–547.
77. Roth A, Sodemann M, Jensen H, et al. Tuberculin reaction, BCG scar, and lower female mortality. *Epidemiology*. 2006;17(5):562–568.
78. Storgaard L, Rodrigues A, Martins C, et al. Development of BCG scar and subsequent morbidity and mortality in rural Guinea-Bissau. *Clin Infect Dis*. 2015;civ452.
79. Kristensen I, Aaby P, Jensen H. Routine vaccinations and child survival: follow up study in Guinea-Bissau, West Africa. *BMJ*. 2000;321(7274):1435–1438.
80. Aaby P, Roth A, Ravn H, et al. Randomized trial of BCG vaccination at birth to low-birth-weight children: beneficial nonspecific effects in the neonatal period? *J Infect Dis*. 2011;204(2):245–252.
81. Hur Y-G, Gorak-Stolinska P, Lalor MK, et al. Factors affecting immunogenicity of BCG in infants, a study in Malawi, The Gambia and the UK. *BMC Infect Dis*. 2014;14(1):184.
82. Black GF, Dockrell HM, Crampin a C, et al. Patterns and implications of naturally acquired immune responses to environmental and tuberculous mycobacterial antigens in northern Malawi. *J Infect Dis*. 2001;184(3):322–329.
83. de Castro MJ, Pardo-Seco J, Martinón-Torres F. Nonspecific (heterologous) protection of neonatal BCG vaccination against hospitalization due to respiratory infection and sepsis. *Clin Infect Dis*. 2015;60(11):1611–1619.
84. Benn CS, Sørup S. Commentary: BCG has no beneficial non-specific effects on Greenland. An answer to the wrong question? *Int J Epidemiol*. 2016;45(6):2131–2133.
85. Ritz N, Hanekom WA, Robins-Browne R, Britton WJ, Curtis N. Influence of BCG vaccine strain on the immune response and protection against tuberculosis. *FEMS Microbiol Rev*. 2008;32(5):821–841. https://doi.org/10.1111/j.1574-6976.2008.00118.x.
86. Biering-Sørensen S, Jensen KJ, Aamand SH, et al. Variation of growth in the production of the BCG vaccine and the association with the immune response. An observational study within a randomised trial. *Vaccine*. 2015;33(17):2056–2065. https://doi.org/10.1016/j.vaccine.2015.02.056.
87. Kandasamy R, Voysey M, McQuaid F, et al. Non-specific immunological effects of selected routine childhood immunisations: systematic review. *BMJ*. 2016;i5225.
88. Netea MG, Joosten LAB, Li Y, et al. Understanding human immune function using the resources from the Human Functional Genomics Project. *Nat Med*. 2016;22(8):831–833.

CHAPTER 8

Epigenetic Rewiring of Monocytes in BCG Vaccination

Rob J.W. Arts, Mihai G. Netea
Department of Internal Medicine and Radboud Center for Infectious Diseases, Radboud University Medical Center, Nijmegen, The Netherlands

Contents

The immune system is typically divided into innate and adaptive immunity. T- and B-lymphocytes mediate the adaptive immune responses, whereas monocytes, macrophages, neutrophils, and NK cells are considered to be the main cellular effectors of innate immunity. It is generally thought that only the adaptive immune responses can build immunological memory, although this property is missing from the cells of innate immune responses. However, this paradigm has recently been challenged. In recent years, there is increasing evidence showing that the innate immune system also possesses adaptive characteristics.[1] Interestingly, in nonvertebrates and even plants, both lacking an adaptive immune system, it has been known for several decades that a memory response can be built, protecting from secondary infections.[2] Interestingly, in contrast to adaptive immune responses, the innate immune memory (named trained immunity) is not strictly specific, as infection with one pathogen often also protects from other nonrelated pathogens.[3]

During the last few years, it was shown that human monocytes and macrophages can build trained immunity after certain infections or vaccinations. When monocytes are exposed in vitro for 24 h to microbial structures such as muramyl dipeptide (MDP) or to the tuberculosis vaccine Bacille Calmette-Guérin (BCG), and a week later restimulated with nonrelated pathogens, they show a significant increase in cytokine production.[4,5] Also in mice, an in vivo challenge with β-glucan protected from a subsequent lethal *S. aureus* challenge,[5–7] and infection with cytomegalovirus improved effector function of NK cells.[8] Looking at older papers from the 1950s and

The Value of BCG and TNF in Autoimmunity
https://doi.org/10.1016/B978-0-12-814603-3.00008-2

1960s, it was shown that vaccination with BCG or comparable mycobacterial proteins[9] induced protection against infections with several pathogens such as *Yersinia pestis,*[10] *Staphylococcus aureus, Salmonella enteritidis, M. fortuitum,*[11,12] *Klebsiella pneumonia,*[13] *Leishmania Major,*[14] *Salmonella enteritidis, Schistosoma mansoni,*[15] herpes simplex, and vaccinia virus,[16] as reviewed in Blok et al.[17] In some experiments, these effects lasted for at least up to a year after vaccination. Furthermore, apart from the effect on lethal infectious diseases, BCG induced potent nonspecific effects during therapy for bladder cancer,[18] other tumors,[19] topical therapy for common and genital warts,[20–22] diffuse cutaneous leishmania,[23] and even as treatment for asthma or type 1 diabetes.[24,25]

Interestingly, comparable effects of BCG vaccination on lethal infections were also observed in human observational data, and later in BCG vaccination trials. It all started with observational data after the introduction of BCG. When BCG vaccination was introduced in the province of Norrbotten in Sweden in 1931, a remarkable drop in mortality was observed. During the first year of life, mortality of BCG-vaccinated children was only 6.6%, yet this number reached up to 22.2% in the nonvaccinated, an effect that was too large to be only the result of the protection from tuberculosis.[26] Furthermore, in 1932, the Pasteur Institute showed, while reviewing their safety data, a mortality of 7.0% among children who had received BCG, compared with 15.3% among nonvaccinated children.[27] As reviewed in Shann,[28] trials also performed in the 1940s and 1950s in the United Kingdom and United States showed a decrease in overall mortality in children vaccinated with BCG; also, an observational trail in more recent years showed comparable nonspecific protective effects after BCG vaccination.[29] Most of these observational studies were performed in Sub-Sahara Africa and have shown that BCG vaccination was correlated with a decreased overall mortality, with mortality rate ratios (MRR) ranging from 0.41 to 0.55.[30–32] Later on, similar analyses have been performed in multiple Asian countries, showing comparable protective effects of BCG.[33,34] To further substantiate the nonspecific effects of BCG, two randomized controlled trials were performed. In the first trial, more than 2000 low-birth-weight children were randomized to receive BCG directly at birth or later on when they were discharged from the neonatal intensive care unit (which is the usual policy). A MRR of 0.49 (0.21–1.15) was shown after 3 days and a MRR of 0.55 (0.34–0.89) after 4 weeks, showing that BCG vaccination increased survival, which could mainly be attributed to fewer cases of fever-related death, for example, neonatal sepsis or lower respiratory infections.[35] Also in a comparable second, but smaller, randomized controlled trial, a same effect of BCG vaccination in neonates was observed.[36] Lastly, a case-control study performed in a similar population also concluded that the BCG vaccine has a nonspecific effect, mainly resulting in a reduction of acute lower respiratory tract infections and infection with respiratory syncytial virus.[37]

To explain these nonspecific beneficial effects of BCG vaccination, two mechanisms have been proposed. The first one is a lymphocyte, and therefore an adaptive immune system-mediated effect, and the second one is trained immunity of the innate immune system that has already been shortly mentioned in the introduction of this chapter. This first mechanism relies on cross-reactivity of T-lymphocytes, which has been named heterologous immunity by others.[38] The mechanisms of heterologous immunity have particularly been well described in viral infections. For example, it ha, been shown in murine studies that BCG vaccination results in protection against vaccinia virus infection through a mechanism dependent on increased T-cell receptor signaling and production of IFNγ by CD4 cells.[39] Interestingly, it has been shown that lymphocyte memory cells can be activated in an antigen-independent manner. Memory cells induced by BCG vaccination can therefore enhance Th1 and Th17 responses upon secondary nonrelated infections, and in this way protect from secondary nonrelated infections.[40–45] It is important to mention the enhanced antibody titer production and T-cell responses to other vaccines such as hepatitis B, polio, and pneumococcal conjugate vaccination after BCG vaccination.[46–48] However, this is not a full explanation for the nonspecific effects of BCG.

The second mechanism is the induction of trained immunity by BCG, a process that completely depends on the innate immune system. In a murine study, it was shown that BCG/PPD-activated macrophages produced more hydrogen peroxide and showed a higher killing capacity of *Candida albicans*.[49] Importantly, SCID mice (that have no adaptive immune system) were also protected from Candida sepsis and showed less fungal outgrowth when they received a BCG vaccination prior to infection. Also, monocytes of these mice showed increased production of TNFα upon ex vivo stimulation with LPS.[4] In another study, B-cell-deficient mice that were BCG-vaccinated showed comparable protection from *S. mansoni* infection as their wild type controls.[50] Vaccination with MDP, a constituent of mycobacterial cells walls that induces trained immunity,[4] results in increased resistance against vaccinia virus and herpes simplex virus in mice. It was also shown that the result was mediated by increased activity of peritoneal macrophages and was not dependent on production of IFNγ.[16]

In humans, there is also evidence that BCG is able to enhance cellular activity. BCG vaccination of healthy volunteers, for example, showed that activity of NK cells was induced.[23,51] When monocytes from cord blood from unvaccinated babies were compared with those of vaccinated infants, an increased expression of perforin and granulysin was shown upon stimulation of these cells.[52] In a trial in West Africa, cytokine production in whole-blood stimulation assays was upregulated in BCG-vaccinated infants.[53] In bladder cancer patients, the amount of M1 and M2 macrophages correlated with the risk of recurrence after BCG installations, which also supports the role of the innate immune system for the nonspecific effects of BCG.[54]

MOLECULAR MECHANISMS BEHIND THE NONSPECIFIC EFFECTS OF BCG ON TRAINED IMMUNITY

The molecular mechanism of how BCG vaccination results in trained immunity and its beneficial nonspecific effects are not completely understood yet. In a first trial, where healthy volunteers were vaccinated with BCG, an increase in proinflammatory cytokine production was observed when monocytes were ex vivo stimulated with *M. tuberculosis*, *S. aureus*, or *C. albicans*. This effect lasted for at least 3 months. When looking at expression of activation markers, an increase of CD11b, TLR4, and CD14 was found. The increased production of proinflammatory cytokines was preceded by increased mRNA expression. Therefore, the hypothesis arose that BCG could induce epigenetic changes in monocytes. It this first trial, occupancy of H3K4me3 was assessed at the promoter sites of *IL6* and *TNFA*, showing an induction of this mark at these promoter sites.[4] As H3K4me3 is a promoter mark that facilitates transcription, this could at least partially be an explanation why more cytokines are produced after BCG vaccination.

In addition, in an in vitro model in which monocytes are trained for 24 h with BCG and restimulated a week later, it was shown that trained immunity induced by BCG was dependent on the recognition by the NOD2 receptor, as monocytes of NOD2-deficient patients could not be trained, and no H3K4me3 changes were induced in these patients.[55] Furthermore, autophagy also appeared to play an important role in the induction of trained immunity by BCG; when autophagy was inhibited, no trained immunity could be induced.[56] Single nucleotide polymorphisms (SNPs) in autophagy genes also resulted in reduced induction of BCG in vitro. Moreover, the same SNPs were correlated with clinical outcome of bladder cancer patients who were treated with BCG instillations, hinting to the fact that the effect of BCG on bladder carcinoma might also be mediated by the innate immune system. To further substantiate the role of epigenetics, induction of trained immunity by BCG in the same in vitro model was inhibited by the addition of the histone methyltransferase MTA.[4] Indeed, the induction of cytokine production a week later was inhibited, showing that epigenetic changes at the level of histone methylation are an essential part of the induction of trained immunity. This therefore proves that the nonspecific memory in trained immunity in monocytes is the result of a rearrangement of the epigenetic landscape of these cells.

Changes in the epigenetic landscape result in better or reduced accessibility of certain genes. Therefore, epigenetic changes in the context of trained immunity in monocytes and macrophages can lead to enhanced cytokine production. Apparently, the rearrangement of the epigenetic landscape results in a more proinflammatory phenotype in trained immunity by inducing epigenetic changes in such a way that mainly proinflammatory genes are more easily translated. So far, the epigenetic assessment has mainly focused on histone modifications, but in non-BCG models of innate immune memory, a role for DNA methylation has been shown.[57,58] Methylation profiles of DNA are a first type of epigenetic change that can be induced in, for example, inflammatory conditions. Cytosine nucleotides of the DNA can be methylated (or demethylated) and thereby the accessibility of DNA by transcription factors is influenced. Methylation of cytosine nucleotides causes genes to become less accessible. This appears to mainly play a small role in innate immune tolerance, where human monocytes are treated with LPS for 24 h and at later time points (up to a week) become unresponsive (thus immunotolerant). However, the amount of genomic regions that are remodeled by cell development from monocyte to macrophage is far bigger,[57] and when specifically assessing DNA methylation remodeling during trained immunity with β-glucan, no specific role for this epigenetic mark could be observed.[57] For BCG-induced trained immunity, no studies assessing the role for DNA methylation have been performed, but given the negative results in β-glucan-induced trained immunity, a major role in BCG-induced trained immunity is unlikely.

A second epigenetic marker that has been more thoroughly assessed in trained immunity are the histone modifications. Histones are the carriers of DNA that efficiently fold DNA to make it fit in the nucleus of a cell. A histone consists of two times four subunits. The H3 and H4 subunits contain a histone tail that can be modified. Several chemical structures can be added or removed by enzymes to specific parts of these tails to change the folding of the DNA and therefore the accessibility of the nearby genes. Two well-known and principally studied chemical groups are methylation and acetylation. Acetylation of histones always results in better accessible DNA. Important examples are acetylation of histone 3 lysine 9 (H3K9ac) or of histone 3 lysine 27 (H3K27ac). Methylation is more complex, as it can both result in better or less accessible DNA, and that depends on the lysine being methylated. Important examples of reduced gene accessibility are histone 3 lysine 9 trimetylation (H3K9me3) or histone 3 lysine 27 trimetylation (H3K27me3). Conversely, histone 3 lysine 4 trimethylation (H3K4me3) facilitates gene transcription. It appeared that histone modifications play an important role in the induction of trained immunity. In a first paper where β-glucan was used to induce trained immunity, major inductions of H3K27ac, H3K4me1, and H3K4me3 were found.[58] When performing pathway analysis on the genomic regions to which the epigenetic changes were allocated, several pathways were revealed important in immune response, chemotaxis and cytokines activity were upregulated, but also several metabolic pathways regulating immune metabolism were induced.[58,59] In a separate paper, it was shown that β-glucan-induced trained immunity also resulted in metabolic changes (the Warburg effect) as a result of induction of H3K4me3 and H3K27ac at promoter sites of glycolysis genes.[59]

For BCG-induced trained immunity, no whole epigenome studies have been performed so far, but based on the studies performed with β-glucan, specifically targeted epigenetic experiments have been performed. First, it was shown that important trained immunity-related genes such as *IL6* and *TNFA* are also epigenetically modified in BCG-induced trained immunity. Induction of H3K4me3 at the promoter site of *IL6* and *TNFA* in monocytes has both been shown in in vitro and in in vivo studies.[4,55] Interestingly, also the inhibitory mark, H3K9me3 appeared to play a role in BCG-induced trained immunity. When monocytes were exposed to BCG in vitro for 24 h, there was a reduction in H3K9me3 at promoter sites of *IL6* and *TNFA* 6 days later.[60] This shows that both a marker that facilitates transcription (H3K4me3) and an inhibitory mark (H3K9me3) are induced respectively removed at the promoter sites of the trained immunity-related genes, resulting in increased production of these two cytokines upon restimulation. This already shows the complexity of the changes in the epigenetic landscape in trained immunity (Fig. 8.1). Second, as described earlier, in β-glucan-induced trained immunity, several changes in immunometabolism were shown to play an important role, and these metabolic changes are induced because of changes in the epigenetic landscape. For example,

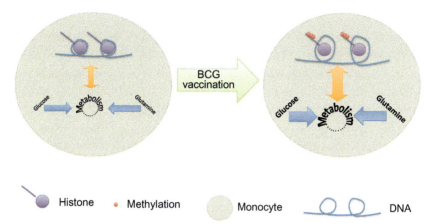

Fig. 8.1 Overview of BCG-induced trained immunity. When moncoytes are trained with BCG, epigenetic changes take place, among others, histone methylation and acetylation, but cellular metabolism is also induced. The epigenetic changes result in higher cytokine production and induction of metabolism. Glycolysis and glutamine metabolism is induced. Interestingly, the induction of metabolism is also necessary for the induction of epigenetic changes, hence, showing a complex interaction between epigenetics and immunometabolism in trained immunity in monocytes.

clear induction of H3K27ac and H3K4me3 at the genomic locations of glycolysis genes were shown.[58,61,62] Accordingly, also in BCG-induced trained immunity, comparable changes take place. Glycolysis is induced, both in vitro and in vivo, and this induction is also the result of epigenetic changes. Again, both an increase of H4K4me3 and a decrease of H3K9me3 are shown at the promoter sites of essential metabolic genes.[63] Interestingly, however, the induction of epigenetic changes is in turn dependent on the upregulation of certain metabolic pathways. For example, if either glycolysis or glutamine metabolism is inhibited, the epigenetic modulations (both H3K4me3 and H3K9me3) at promoter sites of *IL6* and *TNFA* are reversed (Fig. 8.1), hence, revealing a relation between cellular metabolism and epigenetic changes (and vice versa).

This complex relation between the induction of cellular metabolism and epigenetic remodeling at the cellular level has gained more attention in recent years.[64-66] Demethylases and histone methyltransferases are responsible for adding or removing methyl molecules to/from histone tails. Their activity is modulated by several metabolites that serve as cofactors for these reactions. Histone (just as DNA) methylation is modulated by S-adenosyl methionine (SAM), which is derived from the metabolite methionine. It works as a donor of methyl molecules and serves as a cofactor in the methylation reaction.[66] More than 200 genes were predicted to serve as methyltransferases that depend on SAM.[67] However, the exact role of SAM in the induction of trained immunity by BCG still has to be elucidated. Also lysine demethylation enzymes (KDMs) of the JmjC and D family that remove a methyl group from histones depend on α-ketoglutaric acid as a cofactor in demethylation.[68] Interestingly, molecules that resemble α-ketoglutaric acid, for example, other metabolites such as fumarate, succinate, or 2-hydroxyglutarate, operate as inhibitory elements of demethylation, as they interfere with the cofactor α-ketoglutaric acid,[68,69] thus obstructing demethylation, which has already been shown to take place in β-glucan-induced trained immunity.[61] Furthermore, these same metabolites of the Krebs cycle not only interfere with histone demethylases but also inhibit DNA demethylases.[69] This shows the complexity of epigenetic changes and shows that, although no research has been performed on DNA methylation, it is an exciting matter for future investigation.

In conclusion, in this chapter we have shown that innate immunity also has the capacity to adjust by reprogramming the epigenetic landscape of monocytes. We call this *trained immunity* or *innate immune memory*.[1,70] Trained immunity should be seen a new and essential part of the host defense, which induces maturation of innate immune cells of neonates and children after certain infections or vaccinations. Furthermore, trained immunity can be induced in adults, with potential therapeutic applications now being investigated. Nonetheless, we should not undervalue the potential negative effects of trained immunity, with potential roles in the pathogenesis of autoimmune disease or atherosclerosis.[1,71] Hence, increased knowledge of the molecular mechanisms of trained immunity is essential for developing better vaccines, just as for the development of new potential immunotherapeutic interventions and knowledge on how to target inflammatory diseases.[1]

REFERENCES

1. Netea MG, Joosten LA, Latz E, et al. Trained immunity: a program of innate immune memory in health and disease. *Science*. 2016;352:aaf1098.
2. Milutinovic B, Kurtz J. Immune memory in invertebrates. *Semin Immunol*. 2016;28: 328–342.
3. Quintin J, Cheng SC, van der Meer JW, Netea MG. Innate immune memory: towards a better understanding of host defense mechanisms. *Curr Opin Immunol*. 2014;29:1–7.
4. Kleinnijenhuis J, Quintin J, Preijers F, et al. Bacille Calmette-Guerin induces NOD2-dependent nonspecific protection from reinfection via epigenetic reprogramming of monocytes. *Proc Natl Acad Sci USA*. 2012;109:17537–17542.
5. Quintin J, Saeed S, Martens JH, et al. Candida albicans infection affords protection against reinfection via functional reprogramming of monocytes. *Cell Host Microbe*. 2012;12:223–232.

6. Bistoni F, Vecchiarelli A, Cenci E, Puccetti P, Marconi P, Cassone A. Evidence for macrophage-mediated protection against lethal Candida albicans infection. *Infect Immun.* 1986;51:668–674.
7. Kleinnijenhuis J, Quintin J, Preijers F, et al. Long-lasting effects of BCG vaccination on both heterologous Th1/Th17 responses and innate trained immunity. *J Innate Immun.* 2014;6:152–158.
8. Marcus A, Raulet DH. Evidence for natural killer cell memory. *Curr Biol.* 2013;23:R817–820.
9. Williams Jr. CA, Dubos RJ. Studies on fractions of methanol extracts of tubercle bacilli. I Fractions which increase resistance to infection. *J Exp Med.* 1959;110:981–1004.
10. Weiss DW. Enhanced resistance of mice to infection with Pasteurella pestis following vaccination with fractions of phenol-killed tubercle bacilli. *Nature.* 1960;186:1060–1061.
11. Dubos RJ, Schaedler RW. Effects of cellular constituents of mycobacteria on the resistance of mice to heterologous infections I. Protective effects. *J Exp Med.* 1957;106:703–717.
12. Fox AE, Evans GL, Turner FJ, Schwartz BS, Blaustein A. Stimulation of nonspecific resistance to infection by a crude cell wall preparation from Mycobacterium phlei. *J Bacteriol.* 1966;92:1–5.
13. Weiss DW, Bonhag RS, Parks JA. Studies on the heterologous immunogenicity of a methanol-insoluble fraction of attenuated tubercle bacilli (BCG). I antimicrobial protection. *J Exp Med.* 1964;119:53–70.
14. Fortier AH, Mock BA, Meltzer MS, Nacy CA. Mycobacterium bovis BCG-induced protection against cutaneous and systemic Leishmania major infections of mice. *Infect Immun.* 1987;55:1707–1714.
15. Maddison SE, Chandler FW, Kagan IG. The effect of pretreatment with BCG on infection with Schistosoma mansoni in mice and monkeys. *J Reticuloendothel Soc.* 1978;24:615–628.
16. Ikeda S, Negishi T, Nishimura C. Enhancement of non-specific resistance to viral infection by muramyldipeptide and its analogs. *Antiviral Res.* 1985;5:207–215.
17. Blok BA, Arts RJ, van Crevel R, Benn CS, Netea MG. Trained innate immunity as underlying mechanism for the long-term, nonspecific effects of vaccines. *J Leukoc Biol.* 2015;98:347–356.
18. Sylvester RJ, van der MA, Lamm DL. Intravesical bacillus Calmette-Guerin reduces the risk of progression in patients with superficial bladder cancer: a meta-analysis of the published results of randomized clinical trials. *J Urol.* 2002;168:1964–1970.
19. Weiss DW, Bonhag RS, Deome KB. Protective activity of fractions of tubercle bacilli against isologous tumours in mice. *Nature.* 1961;190:889–891.
20. Metawea B, El-Nashar AR, Kamel I, Kassem W, Shamloul R. Application of viable bacille Calmette-Guerin topically as a potential therapeutic modality in condylomata acuminata: a placebo-controlled study. *Urology.* 2005;65:247–250.
21. Nofal A, Yosef A, Salah E. Treatment of recalcitrant warts with Bacillus Calmette-Guerin: a promising new approach. *Dermatol Ther.* 2013;26:481–485.
22. Salem A, Nofal A, Hosny D. Treatment of common and plane warts in children with topical viable Bacillus Calmette-Guerin. *Pediatr Dermatol.* 2013;30:60–63.
23. Pereira LI, Dorta ML, Pereira AJ, et al. Increase of NK cells and proinflammatory monocytes are associated with the clinical improvement of diffuse cutaneous leishmaniasis after immunochemotherapy with BCG/Leishmania antigens. *Am J Trop Med Hyg.* 2009;81:378–383.
24. Faustman DL, Wang L, Okubo Y, et al. Proof-of-concept, randomized, controlled clinical trial of Bacillus-Calmette-Guerin for treatment of long-term type 1 diabetes. *PLoS One.* 2012;7:e41756.
25. Rousseau MC, Parent ME, St-Pierre Y. Potential health effects from non-specific stimulation of the immune function in early age: the example of BCG vaccination. *Pediatr Allergy Immunol.* 2008;19:438–448.

26. Naeslund C. Expérience de vaccination par le bcg dans la province du norrbotten (suède). *Rev Tuberc.* 1931;617–636.
27. Institut Pasteur (Paris France). *Vaccination préventive de la tuberculose de l'homme et des animaux, par le BCG; rapports et documents, provenant des divers pays, la France exceptée, transmis à l'Institut Pasteur en.* Paris: Masson; 1932.1932.
28. Shann F. The non-specific effects of vaccines. *Arch Dis Child.* 2010;95:662–667.
29. Shann F. Nonspecific effects of vaccines and the reduction of mortality in children. *Clin Ther.* 2013;35:109–114.
30. Garly ML, Martins CL, Bale C, et al. BCG scar and positive tuberculin reaction associated with reduced child mortality in West Africa. A non-specific beneficial effect of BCG? *Vaccine.* 2003;21:2782–2790.
31. Kristensen I, Aaby P, Jensen H. Routine vaccinations and child survival: follow up study in Guinea-Bissau, West Africa. *BMJ.* 2000;321:1435–1438.
32. Roth A, Gustafson P, Nhaga A, et al. BCG vaccination scar associated with better childhood survival in Guinea-Bissau. *Int J Epidemiol.* 2005;34:540–547.
33. Hirve S, Bavdekar A, Juvekar S, Benn CS, Nielsen J, Aaby P. Non-specific and sex-differential effects of vaccinations on child survival in rural western India. *Vaccine.* 2012;30:7300–7308.
34 Moulton, L.H., Rahmathullah, L., Halsey, N.A., Thulasiraj, R.D., Katz, J., and Tielsch, J.M. (2005). Evaluation of non-specific effects of infant immunizations on early infant mortality in a southern Indian population. Trop Med Int Health 10, 947–955.
35. Aaby P, Roth A, Ravn H, et al. Randomized trial of BCG vaccination at birth to low-birth-weight children: beneficial nonspecific effects in the neonatal period? *J Infect Dis.* 2011;204:245–252.
36. Biering-Sorensen S, Aaby P, Napirna BM, et al. Small randomized trial among low-birth-weight children receiving bacillus Calmette-Guerin vaccination at first health center contact. *Pediatr Infect Dis J.* 2012;31:306–308.
37. Stensballe LG, Nante E, Jensen IP, et al. Acute lower respiratory tract infections and respiratory syncytial virus in infants in Guinea-Bissau: a beneficial effect of BCG vaccination for girls community based case-control study. *Vaccine.* 2005;23:1251–1257.
38. Gil A, Kenney LL, Mishra R, Watkin LB, Aslan N, Selin LK. Vaccination and heterologous immunity: educating the immune system. *Trans R Soc Trop Med Hyg.* 2015;109:62–69.
39. Mathurin KS, Martens GW, Kornfeld H, Welsh RM. CD4 T-cell-mediated heterologous immunity between mycobacteria and poxviruses. *J Virol.* 2009;83:3528–3539.
40. Berg RE, Cordes CJ, Forman J. Contribution of CD8+ T cells to innate immunity: IFN-gamma secretion induced by IL-12 and IL-18. *Eur J Immunol.* 2002;32:2807–2816.
41. Berg RE, Crossley E, Murray S, Forman J. Memory CD8+ T cells provide innate immune protection against Listeria monocytogenes in the absence of cognate antigen. *J Exp Med.* 2003;198:1583–1593.
42. Hashiguchi T, Oyamada A, Sakuraba K, et al. Tyk2-dependent bystander activation of conventional and nonconventional Th1 cell subsets contributes to innate host defense against Listeria monocytogenes infection. *J Immunol.* 2014;192:4739–4747.
43. Hu J, August A. Naive and innate memory phenotype CD4+ T cells have different requirements for active Itk for their development. *J Immunol.* 2008;180:6544–6552.
44. Lertmemongkolchai G, Cai G, Hunter CA, Bancroft GJ. Bystander activation of CD8+ T cells contributes to the rapid production of IFN-gamma in response to bacterial pathogens. *J Immunol.* 2001;166:1097–1105.
45. Sanger C, Busche A, Bentien G, et al. Immunodominant PstS1 antigen of mycobacterium tuberculosis is a potent biological response modifier for the treatment of bladder cancer. *BMC Cancer.* 2004;4:86.
46. Leentjens J, Kox M, Stokman R, et al. BCG vaccination enhances the immunogenicity of subsequent influenza vaccination in healthy volunteers: a randomized, placebo-controlled pilot study. *J Infect Dis.* 2015;212:1930–1938.

47. Ota MO, Vekemans J, Schlegel-Haueter SE, et al. Influence of Mycobacterium Bovis Bacillus Calmette-Guerin on antibody and cytokine responses to human neonatal vaccination. *J Immunol.* 2002;15:919–925.

48. Ritz N, Mui M, Balloch A, Curtis N. Non-specific effect of Bacille Calmette-Guerin vaccine on the immune response to routine immunisations. *Vaccine.* 2013;31:3098–3103.

49. van 't Wout JW, Poell R, van Furth R. The role of BCG/PPD-activated macrophages in resistance against systemic candidiasis in mice. *Scand J Immunol.* 1992;36:713–719.

50. Maddison SE, Chandler FW, McDougal JS, Slemenda SB, Kagan IG. Schistosoma mansoni infection in intact and B cell deficient mice: the effect of pretreatment with BCG in these experimental models. *Am J Trop Med Hyg.* 1978;27:966–975.

51. Kleinnijenhuis J, Quintin J, Preijers F, et al. BCG-induced trained immunity in NK cells: role for non-specific protection to infection. *Clin Immunol.* 2014;155:213–219.

52. Semple PL, Watkins M, Davids V, et al. Induction of granulysin and perforin cytolytic mediator expression in 10-week-old infants vaccinated with BCG at birth. *Clin Dev Immunol.* 2011;2011:438463.

53. Jensen KJ, Larsen N, Biering-Sorensen S, et al. Heterologous immunological effects of early BCG vaccination in low-birth-weight infants in Guinea-Bissau: a randomized-controlled trial. *J Infect Dis.* 2014;15:956–967.

54. Suriano F, Santini D, Perrone G, et al. Tumor associated macrophages polarization dictates the efficacy of BCG instillation in non-muscle invasive urothelial bladder cancer. *J Exp Clin Cancer Res.* 2013;32:87.

55. Arts RJ, Blok BA, Aaby P, et al. Long-term in vitro and in vivo effects of gamma-irradiated BCG on innate and adaptive immunity. *J Leukoc Biol.* 2015;98:995–1001.

56. Buffen K, Oosting M, Quintin J, et al. Autophagy controls BCG-induced trained immunity and the response to intravesical BCG therapy for bladder cancer. *PLoS Pathog.* 2014;10:e1004485.

57. Novakovic B, Habibi E, Wang SY, et al. Beta-glucan reverses the epigenetic state of LPS-induced immunological tolerance. *Cell.* 2016;167:1354–1368. e1314.

58. Saeed S, Quintin J, Kerstens HH, et al. Epigenetic programming of monocyte-to-macrophage differentiation and trained innate immunity. *Science.* 2014;345:1251086.

59. Cheng SC, Quintin J, Cramer RA, et al. mTOR- and HIF-1alpha-mediated aerobic glycolysis as metabolic basis for trained immunity. *Science.* 2014;345:1250684.

60. Arts RJ, Blok BA, van Crevel R, et al. Vitamin A induces inhibitory histone methylation modifications and down-regulates trained immunity in human monocytes. *J Leukoc Biol.* 2015;98:129–136.

61. Arts RJ, Novakovic B, Ter Horst R, et al. Glutaminolysis and fumarate accumulation integrate immunometabolic and epigenetic programs in trained immunity. *Cell Metab.* 2016;24:807–819.

62. Cheng SC, Scicluna BP, Arts RJ, et al. Broad defects in the energy metabolism of leukocytes underlie immunoparalysis in sepsis. *Nat Immunol.* 2016;17:406–413.

63. Arts RJ, Carvalho A, La Rocca C, et al. Immunometabolic pathways in BCG-induced trained immunity. *Cell Rep.* 2016;17:2562–2571.

64. Donohoe DR, Bultman SJ. Metaboloepigenetics: interrelationships between energy metabolism and epigenetic control of gene expression. *J Cell Physiol.* 2012;227:3169–3177.

65. Hirschey MD, DeBerardinis RJ, Diehl AM, et al. Dysregulated metabolism contributes to oncogenesis. *Semin Cancer Biol.* 2015;35:S129–S150.

66. Kaelin Jr. WG, McKnight SL. Influence of metabolism on epigenetics and disease. *Cell.* 2013;153:56–69.

67. Petrossian TC, Clarke SG. Uncovering the human methyltransferasome. *Mol Cell Proteomics.* 2011;10. M110 000976.

68. Lu C, Ward PS, Kapoor GS, et al. IDH mutation impairs histone demethylation and results in a block to cell differentiation. *Nature.* 2012;483:474–478.

69. Xiao M, Yang H, Xu W, et al. Inhibition of alpha-KG-dependent histone and DNA demethylases by fumarate and succinate that are accumulated in mutations of FH and SDH tumor suppressors. *Genes Dev.* 2012;26:1326–1338.
70. Netea MG, Quintin J, van der Meer JW. Trained immunity: a memory for innate host defense. *Cell Host Microbe.* 2011;9:355–361.
71. Bekkering S, Joosten LA, van der Meer JW, Netea MG, Riksen NP. Trained innate immunity and atherosclerosis. *Curr Opin Lipidol.* 2013;24:487–492.

CHAPTER 9

Mycobacteria, Immunoregulation, and Autoimmunity

Graham A.W. Rook

Centre for Clinical Microbiology, Department of Infection, UCL (University College London), London, United Kingdom

Contents

The Value of BCG and TNF in Autoimmunity
https://doi.org/10.1016/B978-0-12-814603-3.00009-4

INTRODUCTION

There is no doubt that the modern environment plays a major role in the pathogenesis of type 1 diabetes (T1D) and multiple sclerosis (MS). There are low concordance rates (<40% for T1D; <30% for MS) in monozygotic twins,[1,2] and as discussed in greater detail later, the incidences of both diseases increase when people migrate from low-risk to high-risk areas.[2–8] Moreover, environmental factors are increasingly dominant over genetic ones. More cases of T1D are now seen among children who do not have high-risk genotypes,[9] whereas concordance for MS in dizygotic twins is increasing relative to the concordance in monozygotic pairs.[1] Because both are usually thought to be autoimmune diseases where there is a failure of immunoregulation, both have been considered in the context of the "hygiene hypothesis", which suggests that reduced exposure to certain microorganisms early in life might lead to errors in the regulation of the immune system. This hypothesis is beginning to be replaced by the "biodiversity hypothesis" or "Old Friends mechanism",[10,11] which are reformulations of the hygiene hypothesis with more emphasis on Darwinian insights and less emphasis on hygiene.

Enterovirus Exposure

Before discussing the Old Friends mechanism in detail, we need to consider two other factors tentatively implicated in susceptibility to T1D. One suggestion is that modern lifestyles are changing the timing and nature of exposure to enteroviruses, such as coxsackieviruses, and that some of these can trigger autoimmunity. Antibody levels to enteroviruses are diminishing in countries where T1D is increasing, and transfer of protective antibodies from mother to the fetus/baby must also be decreasing.[12] Interestingly, Karelians living in Russia have a much lower prevalence of T1D and allergies than do Karelians living the other side of the border in Finland,[13] and exposure to enteroviruses is greater in Russian Karelians than in Finnish Karelians.[14] Epidemiological studies suggest that certain coxsackievirus serotypes (e.g., CVB1) can trigger and others (CVB3 and CVB6), protect from T1D, prompting the hypothesis that early life exposure to coxsackievirus might be a trigger of T1D, particularly in the absence of maternal antibodies, or if the exposure were at a phase of development that differed from human evolutionary experience. However, several observations cast doubt on the general applicability of this interpretation. First, these studies were performed in families with children carrying an increased genetic risk for type T1D, defined by cord-blood human leukocyte antigen

(HLA) typing,[15] whereas the rise in T1D is not restricted to this subgroup.[9] Second, in the NOD mouse model, coxsackieviruses do not appear to initiate beta-cell autoreactivity; rather, it seems that pancreatrophic serotypes can accelerate the destructive process via a bystander effect if autoreactive cells are already present.[16] Third, children with T1D are at much greater risk for other autoimmune conditions, particularly autoimmune thyroiditis and celiac disease. Indeed, autoantibody studies indicate that, at disease onset, additional autoimmune diseases are already present in approximately one-third of T1D patients.[17] Thus, the overall picture in T1D is of a broad defect in immunoregulation, which fits better with the broad defects predicted by the Old Friends mechanism than with a coxsackievirus-dependent specific triggering event.

Early Life Psychosocial Stressors

A second factor increasingly implicated in T1D is early life psychosocial stress. A large prospective study of >10,000 Swedish children revealed that childhood experience of a serious life event was associated with a significantly increased risk of subsequent T1D, even after correction for genetic factors and other environmental influences.[18] This is interesting because psychosocial stress in early life has long-term effects on immunoregulation and on control of inflammatory responses,[19] which are modulated by microbial exposures (including mycobacteria) as outlined later.[20] Therefore, it is possible to incorporate these epidemiological findings within an hypothesis based upon the Old Friends mechanism.

The Old Friends Mechanism

The Old Friends mechanism suggests that several categories of microbial input coevolved roles in setting up the regulation of the immune system. Therefore, the rising incidences of chronic inflammatory conditions (not only autoimmune diseases but also inflammatory bowel diseases (IBDs), allergic disorders, and some types of cancer and psychiatric disorders) might be at least partly attributable to failing immunoregulation in high-income countries as lifestyle changes deprive us of contact with the Old Friends. This chapter discusses the background to these new interpretations of what used to be called the hygiene hypothesis and reviews evidence that the mycobacteria are significant but neglected components of the Old Friends, with interesting immunoregulatory abilities. Therefore, changed or diminished contact with mycobacteria might constitute an environmental change relevant to T1D, potentially corrected by an appropriate mycobacterial vaccine.

INCREASES IN INFLAMMATORY DISORDERS

The developed countries have undergone massive increases in the prevalence of a wide range of chronic inflammatory disorders including allergies, autoimmune diseases (including T1D and MS), and IBDs. Rigorous meta-analyses that check the diagnostic criteria used have confirmed that these increases are real.[21,22] The increases correlate with economic development and urbanization, and the start of the process in Europe can be traced back to the 19th century when it was noted that hay fever was rare in farmers and characteristic of rich urban educated people.[23,24] Recent studies have confirmed the protective effect of the farming environment[25–28] and shown that contact with animals such as dogs is also protective.[29] A link between lifestyle and an autoimmune disease was explicitly suggested in 1966, when it was reported that the prevalence of MS showed a positive correlation with sanitation in Israel.[30] However, it was not until 1989 that the term "Hygiene Hypothesis" was coined following the observation that, in young adults, a history of hay fever was inversely related to the number of siblings (especially older male siblings) in their family when they were 11 years old.[31] Then, Matricardi and colleagues found that army recruits with evidence of infections attributable to fecal-oral transmission were less likely to have allergic manifestations.[32] Such data were considered consistent with a protective influence of postnatal infection that might be lost in the presence of modern hygiene.[31–33] A few years later it was pointed out that T1D (caused by autoimmune destruction of the insulin-secreting β cells in the pancreas) is increasing at a similar rate, and in the same high-income countries as the allergic disorders.[34] Similarly, a parallel rise in IBDs (Crohn's disease (CD) and ulcerative colitis (UC)) had clearly started at the beginning of the 20th century.[22] Therefore, the original narrow allergy-orientated hygiene hypothesis needed to be expanded and updated to account for diseases mediated not only by Th2 cells, but also by Th1, Th17, or other cell types.[35–37] Similarly, we needed to account for the fact that, as outlined later, the childhood infections were being shown *not* to protect from allergic disorders.[35–37]

Diminished Microbial Exposures and Defective Immunoregulation

Humans coevolved with an array of organisms that, because they needed to be tolerated, took on roles as inducers of immunoregulatory circuits (Fig. 9.1). Such organisms include not only the various microbiotas and commensals (gut, skin, lung, etc.) but also environmental organisms from

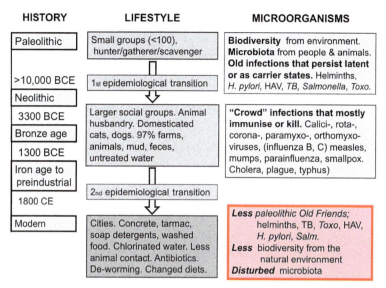

HISTORY | **LIFESTYLE** | **MICROORGANISMS**

HISTORY	LIFESTYLE	MICROORGANISMS
Paleolithic	Small groups (<100), hunter/gatherer/scavenger	**Biodiversity** from environment. **Microbiota** from people & animals. **Old infections that persist latent or as carrier states.** Helminths, *H. pylori, HAV, TB, Salmonella, Toxo.*
>10,000 BCE	1st epidemiological transition	
Neolithic		
3300 BCE	Larger social groups. Animal husbandry. Domesticated cats, dogs. 97% farms, animals, mud, feces, untreated water	**"Crowd" infections that mostly immunise or kill.** Calici-, rota-, corona-, paramyxo-, orthomyxo-viruses, (influenza B, C) measles, mumps, parainfluenza, smallpox. Cholera, plague, typhus)
Bronze age		
1300 BCE		
Iron age to preindustrial	2nd epidemiological transition	
1800 CE		
Modern	Cities. Concrete, tarmac, soap detergents, washed food. Chlorinated water. Less animal contact. Antibiotics. De-worming. Changed diets.	**Less** *paleolithic Old Friends;* helminths, TB, *Toxo,* HAV, *H. pylori, Salm.* **Less** biodiversity from the natural environment **Disturbed** microbiota

Fig. 9.1 Human-microbe coevolution. Humans coevolved with microbiota, with organisms from the natural environment (an unknown number of which contribute to the microbiota), and with certain infections that could persist within isolated hunter-gatherer groups such as helminths and ancient strains of *M. tuberculosis*. These infections had to be nonlethal and were tolerated as latent or subclinical infections or carrier states. Because all these groups of organisms (Old Friends) had to be tolerated, they coevolved roles in driving immunoregulation. The "crowd infections" appeared later after populations increased, but because they kill or immunize, they evolved minimal immunoregulatory roles. Exposure to the Old Friends is diminished after the second epidemiological transition and urbanization. Then chronic inflammatory disorders increase.

animals, the natural environment, and untreated water with which evolving humans were in daily contact, until recently. These "Old Friends" also included infections that were capable of causing stable, chronic, or latent infections, usually picked up at birth and present throughout life.[38] For example, helminthic parasites need to be tolerated because, although not always harmless, once they are established in the host, any effort by the immune system to eliminate them is futile and merely causes tissue damage.[39] *Mycobacterium tuberculosis*[40] and *Helicobacter pylori*[41] are also clear examples of coevolved infections that, in their original form, were in equilibrium with their human hosts. Human exposure to mycobacteria is discussed in greater detail later.

Old Infections Versus Recently Evolved Crowd Infections

Thus the "Old Infections" such as tuberculosis (TB), helminthes, and *H. pylori* that are implicated in setting up immunoregulation (reviewed in Ref. 11) are very different from the "crowd infections" that started to infect man after the first epidemiological transition, when the Neolithic revolution led to agriculture, large settlements, and eventually to urbanization (Fig. 9.1). The "crowd infections" are mostly viruses, like measles, mumps, or rubella (but also diphtheria and pertussis) that could not persist in sparsely distributed hunter-gatherer bands because they either killed the host or induced solid immunity.[38,42–44] Crowd infections need large populations and networks of social contacts so the infection can return to cause an epidemic when herd immunity declines.[38] Such populations did not exist before 10,000 BCE when agriculture and urban development started to allow larger population densities. Some estimates date the arrival of measles in human populations as late as the 11th or 12th centuries,[45] though it might have been earlier, perhaps toward the end of the Roman empire. In the current context, the important point is that humans did not coevolve with the crowd infections, which therefore did not need to be tolerated (they killed or generated solid immunity) so they play little role in setting up immunoregulatory pathways. Numerous large epidemiological studies have confirmed that, and as predicted from these evolutionary considerations, the crowd infections do not protect children from allergic disorders[35–37] and so do not explain the original observations of Strachan that led to the coining of the Hygiene Hypothesis "sound bite". The evidence now supports the view that the crucial immunoregulatory organisms are those previously listed as the Old Friends: microbiotas, Old Infections, and organisms from the natural environment.

Urban Lifestyles and Reduced Exposure to the Old Friends

In conclusion, the current consensus is that the term "hygiene hypothesis" ought to be abandoned, because it is misleading and routinely misinterpreted by the media and the public.[46] The factors depriving modern urban humans of contact with the Old Friends are now well categorized, and hygiene plays a very minor role, except perhaps in reducing exposure to some Old Infections such as helminths. The major disruptor of the microbiota is antibiotic use, particularly in the perinatal period.[47] But diets depleted of plant cell wall polysaccharides often designated "fiber",[48,49] or depleted of plant polyphenols,[50] also lead to less biodiverse microbiota. Moreover, many modern practices such as caesarean deliveries,[51,52] maternal obesity,[53] and lack of breastfeeding impede or distort transmission of the maternal microbiota to the child.[54] Meanwhile, urban dwellers, especially of low socioeconomic status, have diminished contact with the natural environment of which the microbiota seems increasingly relevant to human health.[55–58]

Most of these factors have been explored in relation to T1D, and most do seem to be relevant. Antibiotic use in early life can increase diabetes in NOD mice,[59] but the timing and antibiotic type are critical. Human T1D epidemiology has not yet revealed a convincing link with perinatal antibiotic use, but if timing and antibiotic type are also critical in human babies, this could have been missed.[60] However, antibiotic use *is* associated with a risk of T1D in babies born by caesarean section.[61] Birth by caesarean section in the absence of antibiotic use was associated with an increased risk of T1D in earlier studies[51,62] but not in a very large recent one.[63] Attempts to implicate diet and lack of breastfeeding in susceptibility to T1D are suggestive but not conclusive,[64] but evidence for altered microbiota in T1D is strong and is reviewed later.[65] Indoor dogs increase microbial biodiversity in the home[66] and protect against allergies.[29] Such exposure in the first year of life also protects against developing T1D.[67] This point leads to the issue of the microbiota of the natural environment[56]; this microbiota is particularly rich in mycobacteria, is implicit in much of the epidemiology done on the distribution of T1D, and is discussed in the following sections.

PROGRESSIVE LOSS OF MICROBIAL INPUTS

Does progressive loss of exposure to Old Friends as we modernize and urbanize correlate with increased prevalence of T1D and MS? There are many ways to study this. We can study microbial exposures in the homes of an ethnically and geographically homogeneous population or we can compare urban versus rural populations in the same country. We can also study a genetically homogeneous group living on either side of an international border when the lifestyles in the two countries are very different and document the microbiota of their homes. Similarly, we can study disease patterns within cities in relation to proximity to green spaces. Finally, we can look at the effects of immigration from a low-income to a high-income country. None of these approaches can isolate the effects of diminished microbial exposures from the effects of other exposures (such as the psychosocial stress of immigration), but cumulatively a strong case can be made to support the view that early life microbial exposures modulate the risks of T1D and MS.

The Old Friends Mechanism and Microbial Exposure in a Developing Country

In one remarkable study, all the pregnant women in an area of the Philippines were recruited, and their homes and lifestyle were documented in detail, including the presence and quantity of animal feces in the home.[68] It was found that *high* levels of microbial exposure correlating with exposure to high levels of animal feces in the perinatal period and in infancy correlated with *low* levels of "resting" C-reactive protein (CRP) in adulthood.[68] This was an important observation that helped to explain a crucial paradox. The Old Friends mechanism implies that inflammation is better regulated in developing than in rich urbanized countries. At first sight, this seems absurd because the high prevalence of infections in developing countries might be expected to cause high levels of inflammation.[69] However, recent work by McDade et al. (70, discussed and analyzed in Ref. 71) has largely resolved this paradox. The results reveal that, in a developing country where there is still abundant exposure to the immunoregulation-inducing "Old Friends", immunoregulation is efficient, and the inflammatory response is vigorous during an infection, but it is terminated when no longer needed with the result that "resting" CRP is close to zero. In contrast, in the United States and other developed countries, there is often constant, stable, low-grade inflammation manifested as chronically raised CRP or interleukin (IL)-6 in the absence of any clinically apparent inflammatory stimulus. Such chronically elevated inflammation greatly increases the risk of subsequent inflammatory disease and cardiovascular problems, and has been shown in some studies to predict the future development of depression.[72] Moreover, high serum CRP predicts progression to islet autoimmunity in early childhood.[73]

Urban Versus Rural

Contact with the "Old Friends" rapidly diminishes when industrialization occurs, and individuals start to inhabit a plastic and concrete environment, to consume washed food and chlorine-treated water, and to minimize their contact with mud, animals, and feces. This withdrawal of the organisms that drive immunoregulatory circuits results in defective immunoregulation that, depending on the genetic background of any given individual, can manifest as a variety of chronic inflammatory disorders, including allergies, IBD, and autoimmunity. Early articulations of the hygiene hypothesis focused exclusively on allergic conditions, but we now know that a failure of immunoregulatory mechanisms really can lead to simultaneous increases in diverse types of pathology. For example, genetic defects of the gene encoding the transcription factor Foxp3 lead to the X-linked autoimmunity–allergic dysregulation syndrome (XLAAD) that includes aspects of allergy, autoimmunity, and enteropathy.[74]

The urban > rural phenomenon is also well established for chronic inflammatory disorders and has been explored in some detail in relation to allergies. Contact with the farming environment, whether postnatal[26] or prenatal,[75,76] protects against allergic disorders, whereas the prevalence increases with increasing urbanization.[77] The same is true for IBDs[78,79] and for autoimmune diseases such as MS (Refs. 80,81, discussed in Ref. 82).

Interestingly, T1D is commoner in urban than in rural areas in some countries (Greece, southern Italy, Lithuania[83–85]) but not in others (Finland, New Zealand, or the UK).[86] This might imply that the effect is seen when the comparison is made in poorly developed countries, where rural life is "traditional", with multiple exposures to animals, farm buildings, and soil. A recent study has revealed that rural life only boosts immunoregulation when traditional farming practices are used. This effect is not seen on highly industrialized farms.[28]

The urban-rural comparison therefore suggests either that something beneficial is absent from the urban environment or that something detrimental is present.

Modernized Versus Less Developed; The Karelian Example

Karelia is an area with a rather genetically homogeneous population divided between Russia and Finland. Interestingly, the Finnish Karelians (whose living conditions are considered significantly more modern compared with those of Russian Karelians) have a fourfold higher prevalence of childhood atopy and a sixfold higher prevalence of T1D than the Karelians on the Russian side of the border.[13,14,87] Moreover, the dust in Russian Karelian homes contains far more gram-positive bacteria (mostly Firmicutes and Actinobacteria), 20-fold higher levels of muramic acid, and sevenfold higher numbers of clones of animal-associated species.[13,87] A recent study has revealed that the endotoxin in the guts of Russian infants is mostly derived from *Escherichia coli*, which can protect NOD mice from autoimmune diabetes and drive endotoxin tolerance. But the endotoxin in the guts of Finnish infants is overwhelmingly derived from a Bacteroides species. The endotoxin of this organism fails to protect NOD mice and acts as an *inhibitor* of the agonist effects of *E. coli* endotoxin.[88] Thus it seems likely that one major problem with the "modern" microbiota in Finland is a failure to induce endotoxin tolerance. Consequently, there is reduced immunoregulation, which manifests itself as increases in allergic disorders and in autoimmune destruction of pancreatic β cells, leading to T1D. Importantly, at least three other independent studies have found increased Bacteroides in T1D.[89–91] Indeed, it is clear that the gut microbiota plays an important role in mouse models of T1D,[92] and the same is probably true in the human disorder,[93] as discussed in more detail later.

Age at Immigration

Another way to study loss of microbial exposures is to look at the effects of migration from a low-income to a high-income country. Migration has clear effects on the prevalence of MS, and the crucial events occur very early in life. Iranians who migrate to Sweden have twice the prevalence of MS seen in their birth country.[6] Interestingly, if the second (or later) generation immigrants return to their developing country of origin, they retain their increased susceptibility to MS, which remains higher than in the local population who were not born abroad.[7] A similar phenomenon was seen when people born in the UK (a high MS country) migrated to South Africa (SA: a low MS country). Migration from the UK to SA was protective when the migrant was a child, whereas adult migrants retained their high UK prevalence of MS.[8] Analysis of this and other studies suggests that the environmental factors that protect from or predispose to MS act during the first two decades of life.[4,5]

The same is true for T1D. Here, the crucial factor is to have been born in the receiving developed country, suggesting that relevant environmental factors act very early indeed, or even in the prenatal period.[3] Indeed, the median age at which islet autoantibodies first appear is 2.1 years,[94] though they can first appear at any time between the first years of life[95] and adolescence.[96] The risk of progressing to T1D by 15 years of age correlates with the number of islet autoantibodies present, reaching 79.1% in children with three islet autoantibodies.[94]

Migration also affects IBDs. A definitive study of all first- and second-generation immigrants in Sweden between January 1, 1964, and December 31, 2007, showed that first generation immigrants remain partially protected from both UC and CD, presumably by environmental factors encountered in their countries of origin. However, the diseases increased in prevalence in second generation immigrants, relative to first generation immigrants.[97] Similarly, the prevalence of UC in South Asian immigrants to Leicester in the UK was higher in second than in first generation immigrants.[98] This again indicates perinatal factors.

Sardinia, Malaria, TNF, and the High Prevalence of T1D and MS

Sardinia is an island in the Mediterranean that, since World War II, has developed very high prevalences of T1D and MS.[99] These prevalences make this island an exception to the usual South-North gradient of these conditions. Interestingly, the Sardinians are relatively genetically homogeneous, because they used to hide in the center of the island while surrounding nations contested control of the coastal ports. Malaria was probably introduced to Sardinia by the Phoenicians, perhaps about 900 BCE. Malaria is thought to have spread from gorilla to man in Africa about 10,000 years ago.[100] It then gradually spread into the human populations around the world. Genetic adaptations to malaria varied in different regions (sickle cell disease, thalassemia, G6PD-deficiency, etc). It is suggested that in Sardinia there was selection for variant HLA phenotypes, and for modified control of production of TNF.[99] Interestingly, peripheral blood cells of Sardinian MS patients cultured in vitro did not have more spontaneous TNF release, or more lipopolysaccharide (LPS)-triggered release. But TNF release triggered by malaria parasites was abnormally high.[99] This might be of particular interest in the context of this workshop, because it is conceivable that Sardinians are persistently TNF-deficient in the absence of malaria.

PSYCHOSOCIAL STRESS, IMMUNOREGULATION, AND OLD FRIENDS

Another lifestyle issue is also relevant to immunoregulation and to T1D. Children subjected to serious adverse life events early in childhood develop higher levels of IL-6 in response to a standardized social stressor (the Trier Social Stress Test; TSST) when tested as adults, in comparison to a nonmaltreated control group,[101,102] and maltreated children tend to have higher levels of CRP 20 years later.[103] These observations indicate impaired immunoregulation. Interestingly, negative life events in the neonatal period, whether they affect the child directly or indirectly via traumatic experiences of the mother, also predispose to T1D (Refs. 104,105, reviewed in Ref. 106). This effect of early life psychosocial stress on susceptibility to T1D has been confirmed in a large prospective study of babies born between October 1, 1997, and September 30, 1999, in southeast Sweden.[18] The analysis involved 16,153 children and concluded that the risk of developing T1D before reaching 14 years of age was three times higher in children who had been subjected to traumatic early life events.[18] It is likely that this reflects the influence of perinatal negative life events on subsequent immunoregulation previously described. However, a study of children born in the Philippines suggested that traumatic childhood events did not lead to raised CRP in adulthood in those children who had experienced heavy microbial exposures during infancy.[68,107] In the context of this workshop, it is extremely interesting to note that stress-induced immunodysregulation and a stress-induced chronic inflammatory disorder can be blocked by repeated immunization with a mycobacterium before exposure to the stressor.[20] This issue is discussed later in the context of immunoregulation by mycobacteria.

OLD FRIENDS AND IMMUNOREGULATION

The chronic inflammatory disorders all show evidence of failed immunoregulation (reviewed in Ref. 108). There is abundant evidence that the Old Friends can downregulate the inappropriate immune responses in these conditions. Thus "Old Friends" (such as helminths, nonpathogenic environmental bacteria [pseudocommensals], or certain gut symbionts and probiotics) have been shown to block or treat models of *all* of the chronic inflammatory conditions discussed here.[109–111] This includes the use of BCG to stop T1D in NOD mice[112–114] or to attenuate experimental autoimmune encephalomyelitis (EAE).[115–117] In most cases, the effect has been found to involve conventional immunoregulatory mechanisms. For example, some Old Friends, or molecules that they secrete, can be shown to expand populations of regulatory T cells (Treg)[111,118–120] or to cause dendritic cells (DC) to switch to regulatory phenotypes that preferentially drive immunoregulation.[121,122]

The Old Infections

The most studied of the Old Infections (as defined by Wolfe et al.[38]) are the helminths. As shown in Fig. 9.2, in parts of the world where there was a heavy load of helminths causing immunoregulation, there has been selection for single nucleotide polymorphisms (SNP) or other variants to partially compensate for the immunoregulation[123,124] or to combat new infections such as malaria.[99] This is seen for several proinflammatory cytokines[123] and for IgE production.[124] There is also an increased frequency of a truncated form of the serotonin transporter promoter that has a marked proinflammatory effect.[125] The potential problem here is clear: if the immunoregulation-inducing organisms are withdrawn by the modern lifestyle, these genetic variants might lead to excessive inflammation and become risk factors for chronic inflammatory disorders.[99,123,124]

However, the importance of this phenomenon in modern urban settings is now questionable. In Argentina, when MS patients become

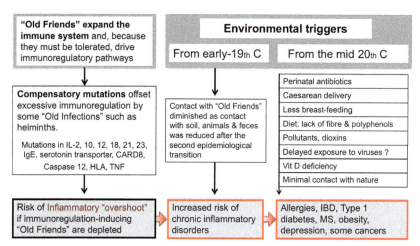

Fig. 9.2 Progressive loss of the "Old Friends". The Old Friends (microbiotas, Old Infections, and organisms from the natural environment) had to be tolerated, so they coevolved roles as triggers of immunoregulatory pathways. In areas with very high loads of Old Friends (particularly helminths), compensatory genetic variants accumulated, to partially restore inflammatory responses. Therefore, when lifestyle changes reduce exposure to the Old Friends, there is increased risk of excessive inflammation, and some genetic variants that were previously beneficial become risk factors for chronic inflammatory disorders. These effects began to emerge when the Old Friends were depleted after the second epidemiological transition and urbanization. More recently, several aspects of modern life are accelerating the loss of exposure to biodiverse Old Friends. The most potent is perinatal use of antibiotics, together with caesarean delivery and lack of breastfeeding. Also of fundamental importance is the distortion of the microbiota due to lack of plant fiber and polyphenols, and reduced dietary diversity. Other lifestyle changes are exacerbating the effects of these changes on the immune system.

naturally infected with helminthes, the disease stops progressing, and circulating myelin–recognizing regulatory T cells (Treg) appear in the peripheral blood,[126,127] indicating that the helminths act as Treg adjuvants. However, when clinical trials with helminths were performed in the United States, results were disappointing.[128] It is possible that the wrong helminth was used in the clinical trials, but one likely explanation is that, despite the selection for proinflammatory SNP in countries with high helminth loads, most of the requirement for the presence of helminths is epigenetically programmed in individuals whose immune systems developed in the presence of helminths that were passed on from the mother in very early life.[129] In fact, the loads of helminths, their location (blood, tissues, or gut), and the mechanisms of their immunosuppressive effects are so varied that is difficult to imagine that an evolved requirement for helminths could have been incorporated into the human genome, and epigenetic effects on the regulation of immune systems that develop in the presence of helminths seem more likely.[130,131] If this is correct, after a few generations without helminth infections in the United States, the presence of helminths might become unnecessary or even harmful.[129]

The Old Infection of particular interest to this workshop—tuberculosis—is considered separately later.

Immunoregulation by the Gut Microbiota

The gut microbiota drive development of the immune system and in particular its regulatory mechanisms.[132] Numerous mechanisms are involved, and these will not be reviewed here. For example, the microbiota releases pharmacologically active components, and metabolites such as short chain fatty acids (SCFA) generated by fermenting dietary fiber (plant cell wall polysaccharides) that cause expansion of Treg populations.[120,133,134] Thus, changes in the microbiota, which is profoundly different in Europeans than in people living in a traditional rural African village,[135] have a major impact on immunoregulation.[132] In the context of this workshop, it is important to note that there is a critical window in early life when the presence of an appropriate gut microbiota is essential for the development of correctly functioning immune and metabolic systems.[136]

Gut Microbiota and T1D

The relevance of the immunoregulatory effects of gut microbiota to T1D is suggested by animal and human studies. The incidence of spontaneous diabetes in NOD mice is quite different in different laboratories, suggesting an environmental variable.[137] The incidence of diabetes is higher in NOD mice housed under pathogen-free conditions than in a conventional animal facility.[138] In agreement with this observation, administration of probiotics to NOD mice reduces the incidence of autoimmune diabetes.[139] More recently it was noted that intestinal type 1 regulatory T (Tr1) cells (IL-10-secreting regulatory cells) can cure T1D in the NOD mouse, and the production of this cell type is strongly influenced by the nature of the microbiota.[140]

Studies of children at risk for T1D and appropriately matched controls reveal that the gut microbiota of diabetic children is different from that of controls.[91,141–144] There is decreased microbial biodiversity and fewer strains that produce antiinflammatory SCFA.[91,141–143] There is evidence for increased infiltration by inflammatory cells in the guts of patients with T1D and a deficit in Foxp3$^+$CD4$^+$CD25$^+$ regulatory cells.[144–146] Correlations between reduced gut microbial biodiversity and poor control of inflammation are a common finding.[147] Gut microbiota of limited diversity is also characteristic of human inflammation-associated conditions such as obesity and IBD.[148,149] Similarly, diminished microbiota biodiversity in institutionalized elderly people correlates with diminished health and raised levels of peripheral inflammatory markers such as IL-6.[150]

Immunoregulation Via the Airways

Microorganisms and other biogenic aerosol materials from the natural environment enter the airways and interact with a number of cellular sensor systems that monitor the content of inhaled air. One of these involves the PI3K/Akt/mTORC1 signaling system that plays a role in inflammatory pathways via NF-κB. Overactive Akt and mTOR (mTORC1) contribute to many pathological processes including cancers, diabetes, inflammation, and neurodegenerative diseases.[151] Natural products from bacteria, algae, fungi, and higher plants can inhibit the activities of these protein kinases.[151] Components of biogenic aerosols from the natural environment also exert antiinflammatory effects via the Aryl hydrocarbon receptor (AhR),[152] and microbe-generated metabolites of tryptophan trigger the AhR, driving production of IL-22, TGF-β, and Treg.[153–155]

A major microbial component in inhaled air is endotoxin (LPS), and the phenomenon known as "endotoxin tolerance" is important in the gut, as previously outlined, but also in the airways. Frequent low doses of LPS trigger epithelial cells via TLR4 and NF-κB, and in addition to a range of inflammatory mediators, drive increased production of A20 (encoded by *Tnfaip3*). A20 is an ubiquitin-modifying enzyme that attenuates NF-κB activation and therefore reduces influx and activation of DC in the airways.[156] Thus exposure to LPS, or to farm dust, blocked a mouse model of allergic asthma induced by house dust mite, and this effect was attributable to A20.[156] LPS did not block induction of asthma in animals that did not express A20 in their lung epithelial cells.[156] Interestingly, a previously unrecognized genetic disorder has been described in human families with an early onset systemic inflammatory disorder. The disease is caused by germline mutations in the gene that encodes A20.[157] The relevance of these observations to humans is strongly suggested by a recent study of two culturally isolated farming communities in the United States. The Amish use traditional farming methods, whereas the Hutterites are industrialized. The Amish have much lower levels of asthma. The study revealed that the traditional farming methods of the Amish expose them to higher levels of LPS in dust. The Amish children have fewer eosinophils in their peripheral blood and more neutrophils. Peripheral blood leukocytes from the Amish have different patterns of gene expression and release lower levels of cytokines when exposed to LPS in vitro. Notably, cells from the Amish children express more *Tnfaip3,* the gene that encodes A20.[28] Thus it is suggested that chronic exposure of the airways to low-dose environmental microbiota (which are then passed to the gut) sets up regulatory pathways within the airways, perhaps systemically. Unfortunately, the prevalence of T1D in these communities does not seem to have been studied, but it is likely to parallel the situation described earlier in the section on "Modernized versus less developed lifestyles", where we noted that induction of immunoregulation via endotoxin tolerance in the gut seems to be a factor in the lower prevalence of T1D in Russian versus Finnish Karelians.

A20 in T1D

The involvement of the *Tnfaip3* gene product A20 in immunoregulation by the natural environment is of particular interest in the context of T1D. A recent study has revealed that, in β-cells, the promotion of survival by A20 is not all attributable to inhibition of NF-κB. A20 also inhibits apoptosis and activates survival signaling in these cells. Thus A20 is antiapoptotic and plays a critical role in the regulation of β-cell survival.[158] Moreover, in children suffering from T1D, the presence of the rs2327832 SNP (SNO) of *Tnfaip3* predicted higher hemoglobin A1c (HbA1c) levels and lower C-peptide levels 12 months after disease onset, suggesting lower residual β-cell function and reduced glycemic control.[158] It is likely that this SNP results in reduced expression of A20, but this is not yet known for certain. Thus a generalized lack of exposure to microbes and to appropriate forms of endotoxin, whether via the gut or via the airways, leading to reduced expression of A20, could be involved in susceptibility to T1D.

Other Immunoregulatory Mechanisms

As previously outlined, there is epidemiological and microbiological evidence to support the view that both human T1D and spontaneous islet cell autoimmunity in the NOD mouse are modulated by microbial exposures that influence Treg and antiinflammatory mediators.[159–162] However, identification of Treg is not always reliable because Foxp3 is expressed in activated T cells. Two alternative regulatory mechanisms have been proposed, and each has been found to be faulty in NOD mice and in human T1D.

First, a novel class of CD52^{hi} CD4$^+$ regulatory cells has been described, and their frequency and function in response to the islet autoantigen, glutamic acid decarboxylase 65 (GAD65), was found to be impaired in children at risk for T1D.[163] These cells were not derived from CD25^{hi} cells and were not Foxp3 positive.[163] These cells release CD52 from their cell surface. This then binds to the inhibitory sialic acid-binding immunoglobulin-like lectins-10 (Siglec-10) receptor on T cells and attenuates effector T-cell activation.[164] It is not known how this new immunoregulatory pathway relates to the Old Friends mechanism.

Second, several findings suggest an immunoregulatory role for TNF. Human TNF was protective against T1D in NOD mice,[165] as was overexpression of murine TNF in the pancreatic islets, despite causing massive insulitis.[166] It has been suggested that this is explained by the ability of TNF to kill human and mouse autoreactive T cells in vitro,[167–169] though some authors suggest that *any* bystander T cell is liable to undergo apoptosis in a site of BCG-induced inflammation, not just the autoreactive ones.[115] Further support for an immunoregulatory role for TNF is derived from the fact that use of anti-TNF can trigger many types of autoimmunity,[170] including MS[171] and T1D.[172]

HUMANS AND MYCOBACTERIA

Is it possible that the immunoregulatory properties of mycobacteria are directly relevant to the increases in T1D? As already suggested, the mycobacteria can be regarded as significant "Old Friends", having been present in the microbiota (see later) and present in the natural environment, and present as one of the Old Infections encountered by evolving humans.

Mycobacteria in the Human Microbiota

The sensitive staining techniques available to clinical mycobacteriologists (Ziehl-Neelsen, or auramine), and more recently immunohistochemistry or in situ polymerase chain reaction (PCR) methods, have resulted in a widespread claims that mycobacteria can sometimes be detected in the gut, oropharynx, or other tissues.[173] However, extracting DNA from mycobacteria is difficult. Recently, the failure of "omics" approaches to find mycobacteria despite their undoubted presence has been highlighted by a study that used drastic methods to break down the tough mycobacterial cell wall. This approach revealed the presence of numerous species of mycobacteria in the oropharynx of all donors investigated.[174] These organisms might not be abundant, but they will be a significant component of the load of bacteria sampled by the lymph nodes of Waldeyer's tonsillar ring, and by the dendritic cells of the small bowel.[175]

Human Exposures to Mycobacteria in the Natural Environment

This problem of extracting mycobacterial DNA also probably explains why most studies of the microbiota fail to report mycobacteria, despite the fact that these organisms are present in the oropharynx[174] and abundant in all soil and many water supplies.[176] Some mycobacteria can be internalized by plants, and up to 10^4/g *Mycobacterium avium* organisms were demonstrated inside plant tissues.[177] Some species, particularly members of the *M. avium/M. intracellulare* complex, can be pathogenic, and even when they do not cause overt disease, they may persist within human tissues. In rural environments, most individuals show skin-test reactivity to reagents prepared from mycobacteria living in their geographical area.[178] Thus, immunologically relevant exposure definitely occurs. Indeed, it has been known for decades that, when mycobacteria are ingested, they rapidly associate with gut epithelial cells and translocate to Peyer's patches.[179] Therefore, mycobacteria will provide a substantial data input to the dendritic cells in the small bowel that sample gut contents.[175]

Modern life must be causing major changes in the balance of mycobacterial species encountered. Intake from water supplies is likely to be maintained but quite different from that encountered by our ancestors. There is a large mycobacterial content in the biofilm in water distribution systems and shower heads, but the species present and their numbers are influenced by the water purification methods used.[180,181] Switching from chlorine to chloramine causes significant changes. In summary, there is no doubt that modern urban humans are still exposed to mycobacteria, but the species, routes, and quantities may be quite different from those experienced by our evolving hunter-gatherer ancestors and strongly influenced by our way of life, our contact with soil, use of showers, and the extent of chlorination or chloramination of water supplies.

Tuberculosis as an "Old Infection" in Evolving Humans

It used to be thought that TB was a recent arrival in human populations, but that is no longer believed. Human-infecting organisms resembling *Mycobacterium canettii* probably evolved in Africa from environmental soil mycobacteria as much as 2.8 million years ago, in which case they might have infected human ancestors as far back as *Homo habilis*.[40] The *M. tuberculosis* complex evolved from these strains in Africa at least 70,000 years ago and accompanied the out-of-Africa human migrations. Ancient DNA and lipid biomarkers have confirmed human TB in a woman and child who lived in what is now Israel about 9000 years ago,[182] and there is both archaeological and molecular evidence that the disease was present in the Americas before historical contacts with Europeans.[40]

An interesting evolutionary hypothesis has been inspired by this long association between humans and *M. tuberculosis.* Meat provides nicotinamide (the amide of niacin; vitamin B3) and also tryptophan that can be converted to nicotinamide in the liver. The nicotinamide is incorporated into NAD and NADH, essential for development and function of the big human brain, and of the immune system. Nicotinamide deficiency leads to pellagra, which is accompanied by inflammatory lesions, mental disturbances, and eventually dementia. Nicotinamide deficiency is often seen with diets dominated by maize or with severe lack of protein. But *M. tuberculosis* secretes nicotinamide, and it has been suggested that subclinical infection with early variants of *M. tuberculosis* provided a backup source of this essential nutritional factor.[183] These early TB strains were necessarily of low virulence, and so able to persist subclinically in small hunter-gatherer groups like the other "Old Infections".[38] More recently, TB has been evolving into a "crowd infection", with increasing virulence, and detrimental effects on life span, but the early strains, probably derived from *M. canettii,* were very different.

Humans therefore probably coevolved with latent TB infection. Even now, about one-third of the world's population is latently infected with *Mtb.* This is readily demonstrated by in situ PCR.[173,184] But such latent mycobacterial DNA is not found in citizens of high-income countries such as Norway where *M. tuberculosis* is no longer endemic.[173] In high-income countries, we are largely deprived of this "Old Friend". Clearly, as discussed later, BCG vaccination might be seen as a way of mitigating diminishing exposure to *M. tuberculosis* and to environmental mycobacteria.

MYCOBACTERIA AND IMMUNOREGULATION

Bacterial components act as essential signals for the development of host tissues, particularly the immune system. These signals are relevant even before birth, as bacterial components, some bound to maternal antibodies, are transmitted to the fetus.[185] Similarly, we know that certain forms of LPS are important drivers of immunoregulation,[88] including expression of A20[156] as previously outlined. However, to my knowledge, nothing is known about the possibility that there are mycobacterial molecules essential for healthy development. *M. tuberculosis* produces a range of molecules that act via the mannose receptor (MR), dectin-2, and TLR2.[186] They also release lipoarabinomannan, lipoarabinomannan carrier protein, Glyceraldehyde-3 phosphate dehydrogenase, Hsp60, and Hsp70 that signal via DC-SIGN.[186] All of these molecules have immunoregulatory properties.[186] Moreover, both *M. tuberculosis* and BCG are well-known to induce Treg.[187,188]

In addition to these mainly *anti*-inflammatory immunoregulatory properties, mycobacteria also contain N-glycolyl muramyl peptides, that prime monocytes via NOD2 to make more IL-1 and TNF.[189] Thus subclinical mycobacterial infections might play a useful role by activating appropriate background levels of innate and adaptive immunity. This concept has been called "Trained Immunity" and might explain the evidence that vaccination with an attenuated strain of a related species, Bacille Calmette-Guérin (BCG), protects not only against tuberculosis, but also against other infections, allergies, and some cancers.[190,191] Increased release of TNF has been postulated as a mechanism that helps to eliminate potentially autoreactive T cells,[167–169] so these N-glycolyl peptides could be relevant in this antiinflammatory context too.

Mycobacteria and TNF

As previously outlined, some auto-reactive T cells in mouse models[168,169] and in man[167] might be driven to undergo apoptosis by TNF. However, in the absence of latent TB (or of other TNF-driving infections such as malaria discussed in the previous section), it is postulated that there might be TNF-deficiency early in life and abnormal persistence of autoreactive T cells. Moreover, it is postulated that BCG vaccination in early life might be able to substitute for *M. tuberculosis* and drive adequate TNF levels. Large intraperitoneal doses of live BCG in mice (10^7 live Connaught BCG[192] or 10^8 Sanofi Pasteur BCG[193]) induced a classical cytokine-mediated sickness response that became chronic and evolved into depressive-like behaviors in 7 days. Not surprisingly, therefore, it was found that these large doses of intraperitoneal BCG in a very small rodent induced impressive increases in plasma TNF levels lasting several weeks.[192,193] But would intradermal BCG in humans cause significant systemic TNF release, and what factors would determine this release?

BCG Trials in T1D

A number of clinical trials of a single dose of BCG in tuberculin-negative individuals with T1D were performed before the year 2000.[194–197] These studies showed no evidence of efficacy. A more recent proof of principle study used two doses of BCG in individuals with long term diabetes and no demonstrable C-peptide, hoping to induce some return of insulin function.[198] Some signs of increased C-peptide were reported, and this study is considered in detail elsewhere in this volume (Chapter 2). There have also been trials of BCG in MS.[199–201] The shortcomings of the earlier T1D studies were analyzed previously.[202] Briefly, small doses of BCG were given to tuberculin-negative donors, and this would be unlikely to induce significant levels of systemic TNF release, or significant systemic changes in Treg, except for those specific for the mycobacteria themselves.[202] It is however possible that these effects can be achieved by using multiple doses of BCG. One preliminary retrospective epidemiological study of only 130 children with T1D compared with 260 healthy children concluded that repeated BCG vaccinations, starting during the first month of life, provided significant protection against development of T1D.[203]

Multiple Injections of Killed Environmental Mycobacteria

An alternative mycobacterial strategy for inducing temporary systemic cytokine release and increased Treg would be repeated injection of a killed preparation of a saprophytic species. Repeated intradermal injections of heat-killed *Mycobacterium vaccae* have been found to be safe in several studies. Five doses were used in a moderately successful trial of *M. vaccae* for the prevention of TB in >1000 HIV-positive Tanzanians,[204] and multiple doses have also been administered in cancer trials.[205] No serious adverse events were recorded. A large body of work indicates that *M. vaccae* works at least partly by inducing regulatory T cells and cytokines.[206–208] However repeated injections can cause sickness behavior, malaise, and influenza-like symptoms suggesting significant systemic cytokine release (own unpublished observations). This might therefore represent a safe way to achieve transiently raised cytokine levels and should perhaps be considered if it is felt that there is sufficient evidence that such levels deplete autoreactive T cells.

More recently, repeated immunizations with *M. vaccae* have been assessed in a mouse model in which a standardized laboratory stressor causes changes to the gut microbiota, behavioral changes reminiscent of depression or posttraumatic stress disorder (PTSD), and colitis.[20] In this model, repeated immunizations with *M. vaccae*, administered before exposure to the stressor, block the behavioral changes, reduce stress-induced changes to the microbiota, and, importantly, block the development of the colitis. These effects were dependent upon the presence of Treg.[20] These observations are of particular interest because reduction of stress-induced changes to microbiota and immunoregulation might be regarded as helpful in the context of T1D, where both early-life stress[18] and microbiota[144] have been implicated. It is entirely possible that BCG used appropriately would be able to exert similar effects.

CONCLUSIONS

The original hygiene hypothesis was a narrow concept suggesting that childhood infections that might be diminished by domestic hygiene are able to protect from allergic disorders. This notion, although based on a pioneering observation,[31] focused attention on the wrong organisms (the recently evolved "crowd infections") and on a minor mechanism (Th1/Th2 balance). We now prefer the terms "biodiversity hypothesis"[10] or "Old Friends mechanism",[129,209] and we see these concepts in the context of the broad spectrum of coevolved interactions between mammals and macro- or micro-organisms, ranging from the endosymbiotic origin of eukaryote organelles, through the microbiota, to true infections. These interactions have numerous functions, many of them metabolic. But we are only just beginning to understand some of the ways in which these interactions regulate our immune systems. In this chapter, I have stressed that mycobacteria will have been present throughout human evolution, and that relatively avirulent strains of *M. tuberculosis* will have been present for at least the last 70,000 years. In fact, mycobacteria were present in all three broad categories of "Old Friends": organisms from the natural environment, microbiota, and Old Infections. These mycobacteria are likely to have driven immunoregulatory mechanisms,[186–190] some of which are listed in Figs. 9.3 and 9.4. These include TNF-mediated apoptosis of autoreactive cells,[167–169] and various aspects of Treg development and survival.[186–189] But mycobacteria are only part of the story. We now understand that reduced exposure to microbial biodiversity in general is detrimental to the immune system. Modern lifestyles reduce and distort our exposure to symbiotic microbiota, to the "Old Infections", and to organisms from the natural environment. This limits the repertoire of the effector arm of the immune system,[210] limits the development of immunoregulatory functions, predisposes to chronic inflammatory states,[129] and increases susceptibility to further immune dysregulation following exposure to psychosocial stressors.[19] Fig. 9.4 is an attempt to express these complex interactions in a simple summary diagram. The yellow stars represent points where we can anticipate that mycobacteria will exert beneficial immunoregulatory effects.

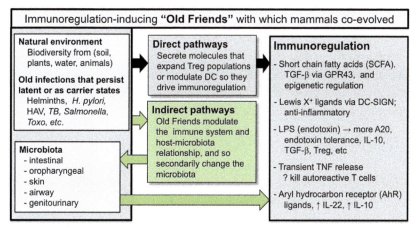

Fig. 9.3 Old Friends and immunoregulation. Some of the Old Friends secrete molecules that directly expand Treg populations, drive release of immunoregulatory cytokines, or modulate dendritic cells so these tend to drive regulatory rather than aggressive responses. Some microbial components such as LPS drive transient inflammatory responses that may eliminate potentially autoreactive T cells, and then, via the mechanisms of endotoxin tolerance, enhance immunoregulatory pathways. However other Old Friends exert their effects indirectly by causing changes to the microbiota, which then secondarily modulate the immune system via a multiplicity of pathways. Some representative pathways are listed in the figure.

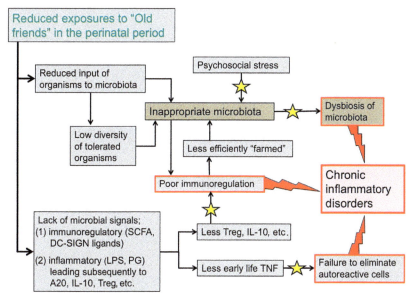

Fig. 9.4 Targets for mycobacterial prevention or therapy. The network of interactions that might predispose to autoimmune disease. The yellow stars indicate points within the network where experimental data suggest that repeated exposure to mycobacteria would be expected to exert a beneficial immunoregulatory influence.

The hypothesis that BCG vaccine could be used in preventative or therapeutic strategies to combat T1D can be viewed in two ways. First, it is not unreasonable to suggest that humans coevolved with mycobacteria and have some evolved dependence on them. If this is correct, then a mycobacterial vaccine might compensate specifically for this loss.

Perhaps more probable is the view that modern humans have multiple deficits in their exposure to microbial biodiversity, and as suggested by some studies previously outlined, a deficit in exposure to the levels of endotoxin required to drive early life TNF release and subsequent endotoxin tolerance and immunoregulation.[28,88] Nevertheless, immunization with mycobacteria might be sufficient to drive immunoregulatory pathways relevant to the increasing prevalence of T1D. Animal experiments with BCG are encouraging,[112–114] and *M. vaccae* is effective in models of allergy and colitis.[20,207] Both organisms are available for human use, and safe when given on multiple occasions. We should not be discouraged by the failure of early trials that used single low-dose BCG in tuberculin-negative T1D. It is clear that, for prevention, we should be thinking in terms of multiple vaccinations, preferably starting soon after birth. For treatment, we need clinical trials of BCG or *M. vaccae* administered on multiple occasions. But in view of the increasing interest in endotoxin tolerance and A20, we should also be considering other interventions such as TLR4 agonists that might drive transient TNF release, and subsequent immunoregulation.

REFERENCES

1. Kuusisto H, et al. Concordance and heritability of multiple sclerosis in Finland: study on a nationwide series of twins. *Eur J Neurol*. 2008;15(10):1106–1110.
2. Knip M. Pathogenesis of type 1 diabetes: implications for incidence trends. *Horm Res Paediatr*. 2011;76(Suppl 1):57–64.
3. Soderstrom U, Aman J, Hjern A. Being born in Sweden increases the risk for type 1 diabetes—a study of migration of children to Sweden as a natural experiment. *Acta Paediatr*. 2012;101(1):73–77.
4. Milo R, Kahana E. Multiple sclerosis: geoepidemiology, genetics and the environment. *Autoimmun Rev*. 2010;9(5):A387–394.
5. Gale CR, Martyn CN. Migrant studies in multiple sclerosis. *Prog Neurobiol*. 1995; 47(4–5):425–448.
6. Ahlgren C, Oden A, Lycke J. A nationwide survey of the prevalence of multiple sclerosis in immigrant populations of Sweden. *Mult Scler*. 2011.
7. Cabre P. Environmental changes and epidemiology of multiple sclerosis in the French West Indies. *J Neurol Sci*. 2009;286(1–2):58–61.
8. Dean G. Annual incidence, prevalence, and mortality of multiple sclerosis in white south-African-born and in white immigrants to South Africa. *Br Med J*. 1967;2(5554):724–730.

9. Penno MA, et al. Environmental determinants of islet autoimmunity (ENDIA): a pregnancy to early life cohort study in children at-risk of type 1 diabetes. *BMC Pediatr.* 2013;13(1):124.
10. von Hertzen L, Hanski I, Haahtela T (2011) Natural immunity. Biodiversity loss and inflammatory diseases are two global megatrends that might be related. EMBO Rep 12(11):1089–1093.
11. Rook GAW. 99th Dahlem conference on infection, inflammation and chronic inflammatory disorders: Darwinian medicine and the 'hygiene' or 'old friends' hypothesis. *Clin Exp Immunol.* 2010;160(1):70–79.
12. Viskari H, et al. Relationship between the incidence of type 1 diabetes and maternal enterovirus antibodies: time trends and geographical variation. *Diabetologia.* 2005;48(7):1280–1287.
13. Kondrashova A, et al. A six-fold gradient in the incidence of type 1 diabetes at the eastern border of Finland. *Ann Med.* 2005;37(1):67–72.
14. Seiskari T, et al. Allergic sensitization and microbial load—a comparison between Finland and Russian Karelia. *Clin Exp Immunol.* 2007;148(1):47–52.
15. Laitinen OH, et al. Coxsackievirus B1 is associated with induction of beta-cell autoimmunity that portends type 1 diabetes. *Diabetes.* 2014;63(2):446–455.
16. Serreze DV, Ottendorfer EW, Ellis TM, Gauntt CJ, Atkinson MA. Acceleration of type 1 diabetes by a coxsackievirus infection requires a preexisting critical mass of autoreactive T-cells in pancreatic islets. *Diabetes.* 2000;49(5):708–711.
17. Triolo TM, et al. Additional autoimmune disease found in 33% of patients at type 1 diabetes onset. *Diabetes Care.* 2011;34(5):1211–1213.
18. Nygren M, Carstensen J, Koch F, Ludvigsson J, Frostell A. Experience of a serious life event increases the risk for childhood type 1 diabetes: the ABIS population-based prospective cohort study. *Diabetologia.* 2015;58(6):1188–1197.
19. Rook GA, Lowry CA, Raison CL. Hygiene and other early childhood influences on the subsequent function of the immune system. *Brain Res.* 2015;1617:47–62.
20. Reber SO, et al. Immunization with a heat-killed preparation of the environmental bacterium *Mycobacterium vaccae* promotes stress resilience in mice. *Proc Natl Acad Sci U S A.* 2016;113(22):E3130–3139.
21. Eder W, Ege MJ, von Mutius E. The asthma epidemic. *N Engl J Med.* 2006;355(21): 2226–2235.
22. Elliott DE, Summers RW, Weinstock JV. Helminths and the modulation of mucosal inflammation. *Curr Opin Gastroenterol.* 2005;21(1):51–58.
23. Blackley CH. *Experimental Researches on the Causes and Nature of Catarrhus Aestivus (Hay-Fever and Hay-Asthma).* London: Baillière Tindall and Cox; 1873.
24. Mackenzie M. *Hay Fever and Paroxysmal Sneezing: Their Etiology and Treatment.* London: Churchill; 1887.
25. von Ehrenstein OS, et al. Reduced risk of hay fever and asthma among children of farmers. *Clin Exp Allergy.* 2000;30:187–193.
26. Riedler J, et al. Exposure to farming in early life and development of asthma and allergy: a cross-sectional survey. *Lancet.* 2001;358(9288):1129–1133.
27. von Mutius E, Vercelli D. Farm living: effects on childhood asthma and allergy. *Nat Rev Immunol.* 2010;10(12):861–868.
28. Stein MM, et al. Innate immunity and asthma risk in Amish and Hutterite farm children. *N Engl J Med.* 2016;375(5):411–421.
29. Ownby DR, Johnson CC, Peterson EL. Exposure to dogs and cats in the first year of life and risk of allergic sensitization at 6 to 7 years of age. *JAMA.* 2002;288(8): 963–972.
30. Leibowitz U, et al. Epidemiological study of multiple sclerosis in Israel. II. Multiple sclerosis and level of sanitation. *J Neurol Neurosurg Psychiatry.* 1966;29(1):60–68.

31. Strachan DP. Hay fever, hygiene, and household size. *Brit Med J.* 1989;299(6710):1259–1260.
32. Matricardi PM, et al. Sibship size, birth order, and atopy in 11,371 Italian young men. *J Allergy Clin Immunol.* 1998;101:439–444.
33. Strachan DP, Taylor EM, Carpenter RG. Family structure, neonatal infection, and hay fever in adolescence. *Arch Dis Child.* 1996;74:422–426.
34. Stene LC, Nafstad P. Relation between occurrence of type 1 diabetes and asthma. *Lancet.* 2001;357:607.
35. Benn CS, Melbye M, Wohlfahrt J, Bjorksten B, Aaby P. Cohort study of sibling effect, infectious diseases, and risk of atopic dermatitis during first 18 months of life. *Brit Med J.* 2004;328:1223–1228.
36. Dunder T, Tapiainen T, Pokka T, Uhari M. Infections in child day care centers and later development of asthma, allergic rhinitis, and atopic dermatitis: prospective follow-up survey 12 years after controlled randomized hygiene intervention. *Arch Pediatr Adolesc Med.* 2007;161(10):972–977.
37. Bremner SA, et al. Infections presenting for clinical care in early life and later risk of hay fever in two UK birth cohorts. *Allergy.* 2008;63(3):274–283.
38. Wolfe ND, Dunavan CP, Diamond J. Origins of major human infectious diseases. *Nature.* 2007;447(7142):279–283.
39. Babu S, Blauvelt CP, Kumaraswami V, Nutman TB. Regulatory networks induced by live parasites impair both Th1 and Th2 pathways in patent lymphatic filariasis: implications for parasite persistence. *J Immunol.* 2006;176(5):3248–3256.
40. Galagan JE. Genomic insights into tuberculosis. *Nat Rev Genet.* 2014;15(5):307–320.
41. Linz B, et al. An African origin for the intimate association between humans and *Helicobacter pylori. Nature.* 2007;445(7130):915–918.
42. Bartlett MS. The critical community size for measles in the United States. *J R Stat Soc Ser A (Gen).* 1960;123(1):37–44.
43. Black FL. Measles endemicity in insular populations: critical community size and its evolutionary implication. *J Theor Biol.* 1966;11(2):207–211.
44. Sharland M, et al. *Manual of Childhood Infections: The Blue Book.* Oxford university Press; 2016.
45. Furuse Y, Suzuki A, Oshitani H. Origin of measles virus: divergence from rinderpest virus between the 11th and 12th centuries. *Virol J.* 2010;7:52.
46. Bloomfield SF, et al. Time to abandon the hygiene hypothesis: new perspectives on allergic disease, the human microbiome, infectious disease prevention and the role of targeted hygiene. *Perspect Public Health.* 2016;136(4):213–224.
47. Blaser MJ. Antibiotic use and its consequences for the normal microbiome. *Science.* 2016;352(6285):544–545.
48. Thorburn AN, Macia L, Mackay CR. Diet, metabolites, and "western-lifestyle" inflammatory diseases. *Immunity.* 2014;40(6):833–842.
49. Sonnenburg ED, et al. Diet-induced extinctions in the gut microbiota compound over generations. *Nature.* 2016;529(7585):212–215.
50. Cuervo A, et al. Phenolic compounds from red wine and coffee are associated with specific intestinal microorganisms in allergic subjects. *Food Funct.* 2016;7(1):104–109.
51. Cardwell CR, et al. Caesarean section is associated with an increased risk of childhood-onset type 1 diabetes mellitus: a meta-analysis of observational studies. *Diabetologia.* 2008;51(5):726–735.
52. Blustein J, et al. Association of caesarean delivery with child adiposity from age 6 weeks to 15 years. *Int J Obes (Lond).* 2013;37(7):900–906.
53. Galley JD, Bailey M, Kamp Dush C, Schoppe-Sullivan S, Christian LM. Maternal obesity is associated with alterations in the gut microbiome in toddlers. *PLoS One.* 2014;9(11):e113026.

54. Pannaraj PS, et al. Association between breast milk bacterial communities and establishment and development of the infant gut microbiome. *JAMA Pediatr.* 2017;171(7):647–654.
55. Mitchell R, Popham F. Effect of exposure to natural environment on health inequalities: an observational population study. *Lancet.* 2008;372(9650):1655–1660.
56. Rook GA. Regulation of the immune system by biodiversity from the natural environment: an ecosystem service essential to health. *Proc Natl Acad Sci U S A.* 2013;110(46):18360–18367.
57. Browne HP, et al. Culturing of 'unculturable' human microbiota reveals novel taxa and extensive sporulation. *Nature.* 2016;533(7604):543–546.
58. Flandroy L, et al. The impact of human activities and lifestyles on the interlinked microbiota and health of humans and of ecosystems. *Sci Total Environ.* 2018;627:1018–1038.
59. Livanos AE, et al. Antibiotic-mediated gut microbiome perturbation accelerates development of type 1 diabetes in mice. *Nat Microbiol.* 2016;1(11):16140.
60. Gulden E, Wong FS, Wen L. The gut microbiota and type 1 diabetes. *Clin Immunol.* 2015;159(2):143–153.
61. Clausen TD, et al. Broad-spectrum antibiotic treatment and subsequent childhood type 1 diabetes: a Nationwide Danish cohort study. *PLoS One.* 2016;11(8):e0161654.
62. Bonifacio E, Warncke K, Winkler C, Wallner M, Ziegler AG. Cesarean section and interferon-induced helicase gene polymorphisms combine to increase childhood type 1 diabetes risk. *Diabetes.* 2011;60(12):3300–3306.
63. Clausen TD, et al. Prelabor cesarean section and risk of childhood type 1 diabetes: a Nationwide register-based cohort study. *Epidemiology.* 2016;27(4):547–555.
64. Nucci AM, Virtanen SM, Becker DJ. Infant feeding and timing of complementary foods in the development of type 1 diabetes. *Curr Diab Rep.* 2015;15(9):62.
65. Paun A, Yau C, Danska JS. The influence of the microbiome on type 1 diabetes. *J Immunol.* 2017;198(2):590–595.
66. Fujimura KE, et al. Man's best friend? The effect of pet ownership on house dust microbial communities. *J Allergy Clin Immunol 126(2).* 2010;126(2):410–412. 412 e411-413.
67. Virtanen SM, et al. Microbial exposure in infancy and subsequent appearance of type 1 diabetes mellitus-associated autoantibodies: a cohort study. *JAMA Pediatr.* 2014;168(8):755–763.
68. McDade TW, Rutherford J, Adair L, Kuzawa CW. Early origins of inflammation: microbial exposures in infancy predict lower levels of C-reactive protein in adulthood. *Proc Biol Sci.* 2010;277(1684):1129–1137.
69. Gurven M, Kaplan H, Winking J, Finch C, Crimmins EM. Aging and inflammation in two epidemiological worlds. *J Gerontol A Biol Sci Med Sci.* 2008;63(2):196–199.
70. McDade TW, et al. Analysis of variability of high sensitivity C-reactive protein in lowland Ecuador reveals no evidence of chronic low-grade inflammation. *Am J Hum Biol.* 2012;24(5):675–681.
71. Rook G, Raison CL, Lowry CA. Childhood microbial experience, immunoregulation, inflammation and adult susceptibility to psychosocial stressors and depression in rich and poor countries. *Evol Med Publ Health.* 2013;2013(1):14–17.
72. Gimeno D, et al. Associations of C-reactive protein and interleukin-6 with cognitive symptoms of depression: 12-year follow-up of the Whitehall II study. *Psychol Med.* 2009;39(3):413–423.
73. Chase HP, et al. Elevated C-reactive protein levels in the development of type 1 diabetes. *Diabetes.* 2004;53(10):2569–2573.
74. Wildin RS, Smyk-Pearson S, Filipovich AH. Clinical and molecular features of the immunodysregulation, polyendocrinopathy, enteropathy, X linked (IPEX) syndrome. *J Med Genet.* 2002;39(8):537–545.
75. Ege MJ, et al. Prenatal exposure to a farm environment modifies atopic sensitization at birth. *J Allergy Clin Immunol.* 2008;122(2):407–412. 412 e401-404.

76. Schaub B, et al. Maternal farm exposure modulates neonatal immune mechanisms through regulatory T cells. *J Allergy Clin Immunol.* 2009;123(4). 774–782.e775.

77. Nicolaou N, Siddique N, Custovic A. Allergic disease in urban and rural populations: increasing prevalence with increasing urbanization. *Allergy.* 2005;60(11):1357–1360.

78. Hou JK, El-Serag H, Thirumurthi S. Distribution and manifestations of inflammatory bowel disease in Asians, Hispanics, and African Americans: a systematic review. *Am J Gastroenterol.* 2009;104(8):2100–2109.

79. Benchimol EI, et al. Rural and urban residence during early life is associated with a lower risk of inflammatory bowel disease: a population-based inception and birth cohort study. *Am J Gastroenterol.* 2017;112:1412–1422.

80. Beebe GW, Kurtzke JF, Kurland LT, Auth TL, Nagler B. Studies on the natural history of multiple sclerosis. 3. Epidemiologic analysis of the army experience in world war II. *Neurology.* 1967;17(1):1–17.

81. Antonovsky A, et al. Epidemiologic study of multiple sclerosis in Israel. I. An overall review of methods and findings. *Arch Neurol.* 1965;13:183–193.

82. Lowis GW. The social epidemiology of multiple sclerosis. *Sci Total Environ.* 1990;90: 163–190.

83. Cherubini V, et al. Large incidence variation of type I diabetes in Central-Southern Italy 1990–1995: lower risk in rural areas. *Diabetologia.* 1999;42(7):789–792.

84. Dacou-Voutetakis C, Karavanaki K, Tsoka-Gennatas H. National data on the epidemiology of IDDM in Greece. Cases diagnosed in 1992. Hellenic Epidemiology Study Group. *Diabetes Care.* 1995;18(4):552–554.

85. Pundziute-Lycka A, Urbonaite B, Ostrauskas R, Zalinkevicius R, Dahlquist GG. Incidence of type 1 diabetes in Lithuanians aged 0–39 years varies by the urban-rural setting, and the time change differs for men and women during 1991–2000. *Diabetes Care.* 2003;26(3):671–676.

86. Miller LJ, et al. Urban-Rural Variation in Childhood Type 1 Diabetes Incidence in Canterbury, New Zealand, 1980-2004. In: *Health Place.* 2010.

87. Pakarinen J, et al. Predominance of Gram-positive bacteria in house dust in the low-allergy risk Russian Karelia. *Environ Microbiol.* 2008;10(12):3317–3325.

88. Vatanen T, et al. Variation in microbiome LPS immunogenicity contributes to autoimmunity in humans. *Cell.* 2016;165(4):842–853.

89. Davis-Richardson AG, et al. Bacteroides dorei dominates gut microbiome prior to autoimmunity in Finnish children at high risk for type 1 diabetes. *Front Microbiol.* 2014;5:678.

90. Alkanani AK, et al. Alterations in intestinal microbiota correlate with susceptibility to type 1 diabetes. *Diabetes.* 2015;64(10):3510–3520.

91. de Goffau MC, et al. Fecal microbiota composition differs between children with beta-cell autoimmunity and those without. *Diabetes.* 2013;62(4):1238–1244.

92. Costa FR, et al. Gut microbiota translocation to the pancreatic lymph nodes triggers NOD2 activation and contributes to T1D onset. *J Exp Med.* 2016;213(7):1223–1239.

93. Knip M, Siljander H. The role of the intestinal microbiota in type 1 diabetes mellitus. *Nat Rev Endocrinol.* 2016;12(3):154–167.

94. Ziegler AG, et al. Seroconversion to multiple islet autoantibodies and risk of progression to diabetes in children. *JAMA.* 2013;309(23):2473–2479.

95. Couper JJ, et al. Weight gain in early life predicts risk of islet autoimmunity in children with a first-degree relative with type 1 diabetes. *Diabetes Care.* 2009;32(1):94–99.

96. Colman PG, et al. Development of autoantibodies to islet antigens during childhood: implications for preclinical type 1 diabetes screening. *Pediatr Diabetes.* 2002;3(3):144–148.

97. Li X, Sundquist J, Hemminki K, Sundquist K. Risk of inflammatory bowel disease in first- and second-generation immigrants in Sweden: a nationwide follow-up study. *Inflamm Bowel Dis.* 2011;17(8):1784–1791.

98. Carr I, Mayberry JF. The effects of migration on ulcerative colitis: a three-year prospective study among Europeans and first- and second- generation south Asians in Leicester (1991–1994). *Am J Gastroenterol.* 1999;94(10):2918–2922.

99. Sotgiu S, Angius A, Embry A, Rosati G, Musumeci S. Hygiene hypothesis: innate immunity, malaria and multiple sclerosis. *Med Hypotheses.* 2008;70(4):819–825.

100. Liu W, et al. Origin of the human malaria parasite plasmodium falciparum in gorillas. *Nature.* 2010;467(7314):420–425.

101. Carpenter LL, et al. Association between plasma IL-6 response to acute stress and early-life adversity in healthy adults. *Neuropsychopharmacology.* 2010;35(13):2617–2623.

102. Pace TW, et al. Increased stress-induced inflammatory responses in male patients with major depression and increased early life stress. *Am J Psychiatry.* 2006;163(9): 1630–1633.

103. Danese A, Pariante CM, Caspi A, Taylor A, Poulton R. Childhood maltreatment predicts adult inflammation in a life-course study. *Proc Natl Acad Sci U S A.* 2007;104(4): 1319–1324.

104. Sepa A, Frodi A, Ludvigsson J. Mothers' experiences of serious life events increase the risk of diabetes-related autoimmunity in their children. *Diabetes Care.* 2005;28(10):2394–2399.

105. Vlajinac H, et al. The Belgrade childhood diabetes study—comparison of children with type 1 diabetes with their siblings. *Paediatr Perinat Epidemiol.* 2006;20(3):238–243.

106. Peng H, Hagopian W. Environmental factors in the development of type 1 diabetes. *Rev Endocr Metab Disord.* 2006;7(3):149–162.

107. McDade TW. Early environments and the ecology of inflammation. *Proc Natl Acad Sci U S A.* 2012;109(Suppl 2):17281–17288.

108. Rook GAW. The broader implications of the hygiene hypothesis. *Immunology.* 2009;126:3–11.

109. Round JL, Mazmanian SK. The gut microbiota shapes intestinal immune responses during health and disease. *Nat Rev Immunol.* 2009;9(5):313–323.

110. Osada Y, Kanazawa T. Parasitic helminths: new weapons against immunological disorders. *J Biomed Biotechnol.* 2010;2010:743–758.

111. Karimi K, Inman MD, Bienenstock J, Forsythe P. Lactobacillus reuteri-induced regulatory T cells protect against an allergic airway response in mice. *Am J Respir Crit Care Med.* 2009;179(3):186–193.

112. Shehadeh N, et al. Repeated BCG vaccination is more effective than a single dose in preventing diabetes in non-obese diabetic (NOD) mice. *Isr J Med Sci.* 1997;33(11): 711–715.

113. Qin HY, Singh B. BCG vaccination prevents insulin-dependent diabetes mellitus (IDDM) in NOD mice after disease acceleration with cyclophosphamide. *J Autoimmun.* 1997;10(3):271–278.

114. Harada M, Kishimoto Y, Makino S. Prevention of overt diabetes and insulitis in NOD mice by a single BCG vaccination. *Diabetes Res Clin Pract.* 1990;8(2):85–89.

115. O'Connor RA, Wittmer S, Dalton DK. Infection-induced apoptosis deletes bystander CD4[+] T cells: a mechanism for suppression of autoimmunity during BCG infection. *J Autoimmun.* 2005;24(2):93–100.

116. Sewell DL, et al. Infection with *Mycobacterium bovis* BCG diverts traffic of myelin oligodendroglial glycoprotein autoantigen-specific T cells away from the central nervous system and ameliorates experimental autoimmune encephalomyelitis. *Clin Diagn Lab Immunol.* 2003;10(4):564–572.

117. Lee J, Reinke EK, Zozulya AL, Sandor M, Fabry Z. *Mycobacterium bovis* bacille Calmette-Guerin infection in the CNS suppresses experimental autoimmune encephalomyelitis and Th17 responses in an IFN-gamma-independent manner. *J Immunol.* 2008;181(9):6201–6212.

118. Round JL, et al. The Toll-like receptor 2 pathway establishes colonization by a commensal of the human microbiota. *Science*. 2011;332(6032):974–977.
119. Grainger JR, et al. Helminth secretions induce de novo T cell Foxp3 expression and regulatory function through the TGF-beta pathway. *J Exp Med*. 2010;207(11):2331–2341.
120. Atarashi K, et al. Induction of colonic regulatory T cells by indigenous Clostridium species. *Science*. 2011;331:337–341.
121. Smits HH, et al. Selective probiotic bacteria induce IL-10-producing regulatory T cells in vitro by modulating dendritic cell function through dendritic cell-specific intercellular adhesion molecule 3-grabbing nonintegrin. *J Allergy Clin Immunol*. 2005;115(6):1260–1267.
122. Hart AL, et al. Modulation of human dendritic cell phenotype and function by probiotic bacteria. *Gut*. 2004;53(11):1602–1609.
123. Fumagalli M, et al. Parasites represent a major selective force for interleukin genes and shape the genetic predisposition to autoimmune conditions. *J Exp Med*. 2009;206(6):1395–1408.
124. Barnes KC, Grant AV, Gao P. A review of the genetic epidemiology of resistance to parasitic disease and atopic asthma: common variants for common phenotypes? *Curr Opin Allergy Clin Immunol*. 2005;5(5):379–385.
125. Fredericks CA, et al. Healthy young women with serotonin transporter SS polymorphism show a pro-inflammatory bias under resting and stress conditions. *Brain Behav Immun*. 2010;24:350–357.
126. Correale J, Farez M. Association between parasite infection and immune responses in multiple sclerosis. *Ann Neurol*. 2007;61(2):97–108.
127. Correale J, Farez MF. The impact of parasite infections on the course of multiple sclerosis. *J Neuroimmunol*. 2011;233(1–2):6–11.
128. Fleming J, et al. Clinical trial of helminth-induced immunomodulatory therapy (HINT 2) in relapsing-remitting MS. *Neurol Poster*. 2014;P3:149.
129. Rook G, Bäckhed F, Levin BR, McFall-Ngai MJ, McLean AR. Evolution, human-microbe interactions, and life history plasticity. *Lancet*. 2017;390(10093):521–530.
130. Report of a WHO Expert Committee. *Prevention and Control of Intestinal Parasitic Infections*. World Health Organization; 1987. Technical Report Series 749.
131. Reynolds LA, Finlay BB, Maizels RM. Cohabitation in the intestine: interactions among helminth parasites, bacterial microbiota, and host immunity. *J Immunol*. 2015;195(9):4059–4066.
132. Levy M, Thaiss CA, Elinav E. Metabolites: messengers between the microbiota and the immune system. *Genes Dev*. 2016;30(14):1589–1597.
133. Round JL, Mazmanian SK. Inducible Foxp3$^+$ regulatory T-cell development by a commensal bacterium of the intestinal microbiota. *Proc Natl Acad Sci U S A*. 2010;107(27):12204–12209.
134. Tan J, et al. Dietary fiber and bacterial SCFA enhance oral tolerance and protect against food allergy through diverse cellular pathways. *Cell Rep*. 2016;15(12):2809–2824.
135. De Filippo C, et al. Impact of diet in shaping gut microbiota revealed by a comparative study in children from Europe and rural Africa. *Proc Natl Acad Sci U S A*. 2010;107(33):14691–14696.
136. Cox LM, et al. Altering the intestinal microbiota during a critical developmental window has lasting metabolic consequences. *Cell*. 2014;158(4):705–721.
137. Pozzilli P, Signore A, Williams AJ, Beales PE. NOD mouse colonies around the world—recent facts and figures. *Immunol Today*. 1993;14(5):193–196.
138. Funda DP, Fundova P, Harrison LC. In: Sanjeevi CB, Gale EM, eds. *Environmental-mucosal interactions in the natural history of type 1 diabetes: the germ-free (GF) NOD mouse model. Proceedings of the 7th Immunology of Diabetes Society Meeting*; vol. 41. New York: Ann N Y Acad Sci; 2005.

139. Calcinaro F, et al. Oral probiotic administration induces interleukin-10 production and prevents spontaneous autoimmune diabetes in the non-obese diabetic mouse. *Diabetologia.* 2005;48(8):1565–1575.

140. Yu H, et al. Intestinal type 1 regulatory T cells migrate to periphery to suppress diabetogenic T cells and prevent diabetes development. *Proc Natl Acad Sci USA.* 2017;114:10443–10448.

141. Brown CT, et al. Gut microbiome metagenomics analysis suggests a functional model for the development of autoimmunity for type 1 diabetes. *PLoS One.* 2011;6(10):e25792.

142. Giongo A, et al. Toward defining the autoimmune microbiome for type 1 diabetes. *ISME J.* 2011;5(1):82–91.

143. Kostic AD, et al. The dynamics of the human infant gut microbiome in development and in progression toward type 1 diabetes. *Cell Host Microbe.* 2015;17(2):260–273.

144. Pellegrini S, et al. Duodenal mucosa of patients with type 1 diabetes shows distinctive inflammatory profile and microbiota. *J Clin Endocrinol Metab.* 2017;102(5):1468–1477.

145. Tiittanen M, Westerholm-Ormio M, Verkasalo M, Savilahti E, Vaarala O. Infiltration of forkhead box P3-expressing cells in small intestinal mucosa in coeliac disease but not in type 1 diabetes. *Clin Exp Immunol.* 2008;152(3):498–507.

146. Badami E, et al. Defective differentiation of regulatory FoxP3$^+$T cells by small-intestinal dendritic cells in patients with type 1 diabetes. *Diabetes.* 2011;60(8):2120–2124.

147. Hildebrand F, et al. Inflammation-associated enterotypes, host genotype, cage and inter-individual effects drive gut microbiota variation in common laboratory mice. *Genome Biol.* 2013;14(1):R4.

148. Turnbaugh PJ, et al. A core gut microbiome in obese and lean twins. *Nature.* 2009;457(7228):480–484.

149. Rehman A, et al. Transcriptional activity of the dominant gut mucosal microbiota in chronic inflammatory bowel disease patients. *J Med Microbiol.* 2010;59(Pt 9):1114–1122.

150. Claesson MJ, et al. Gut microbiota composition correlates with diet and health in the elderly. *Nature.* 2012;488(7410):178–184.

151. Moore MN. Do airborne biogenic chemicals interact with the PI3K/Akt/mTOR cell signalling pathway to benefit human health and wellbeing in rural and coastal environments? *Environ Res.* 2015;140:65–75.

152. Mohammadi-Bardbori A, Bengtsson J, Rannug U, Rannug A, Wincent E. Quercetin, resveratrol, and curcumin are indirect activators of the aryl hydrocarbon receptor (AHR). *Chem Res Toxicol.* 2012;25(9):1878–1884.

153. Zelante T, et al. Tryptophan feeding of the IDO1-AhR Axis in host-microbial symbiosis. *Front Immunol.* 2014;5:640.

154. Bessede A, et al. Aryl hydrocarbon receptor control of a disease tolerance defence pathway. *Nature.* 2014;511(7508):184–190.

155. Quintana FJ, et al. Control of T(reg) and T(H)17 cell differentiation by the aryl hydrocarbon receptor. *Nature.* 2008;453(7191):65–71.

156. Schuijs MJ, et al. Farm dust and endotoxin protect against allergy through A20 induction in lung epithelial cells. *Science.* 2015;349(6252):1106–1110.

157. Zhou Q, et al. Loss-of-function mutations in TNFAIP3 leading to A20 haploinsufficiency cause an early-onset autoinflammatory disease. *Nat Genet.* 2016;48(1):67–73.

158. Fukaya M, et al. A20 inhibits beta-cell apoptosis by multiple mechanisms and predicts residual beta-cell function in type 1 diabetes. *Mol Endocrinol.* 2016;30(1):48–61.

159. Johnson MC, et al. Beta cell-specific IL-2 therapy increases islet Foxp3$^+$Treg and suppresses type 1 diabetes in NOD mice. *Diabetes.* 2013.

160. Pop SM, Wong CP, Culton DA, Clarke SH, Tisch R. Single cell analysis shows decreasing FoxP3 and TGFbeta1 coexpressing CD4$^+$CD25$^+$ regulatory T cells during autoimmune diabetes. *J Exp Med.* 2005;201(8):1333–1346.

161. Haseda F, Imagawa A, Murase-Mishiba Y, Terasaki J, Hanafusa T. CD4(+) CD45RA(−) FoxP3high activated regulatory T cells are functionally impaired and related to residual insulin-secreting capacity in patients with type 1 diabetes. *Clin Exp Immunol.* 2013;173(2):207–216.

162. Harrison LC, et al. Antigen-based vaccination and prevention of type 1 diabetes. *Curr Diab Rep.* 2013;13(5):616–623.

163. Bandala-Sanchez E, et al. T cell regulation mediated by interaction of soluble CD52 with the inhibitory receptor Siglec-10. *Nat Immunol.* 2013;14(7):741–748.

164. Toh BH, Kyaw T, Tipping P, Bobik A. Immune regulation by CD52-expressing CD4 T cells. *Cell Mol Immunol.* 2013.

165. Satoh J, et al. Recombinant human tumor necrosis factor alpha suppresses autoimmune diabetes in nonobese diabetic mice. *J Clin Invest.* 1989;84(4):1345–1348.

166. Grewal IS, et al. Local expression of transgene encoded TNF alpha in islets prevents autoimmune diabetes in nonobese diabetic (NOD) mice by preventing the development of auto-reactive islet-specific T cells. *J Exp Med.* 1996;184(5):1963–1974.

167. Ban L, et al. Selective death of autoreactive T cells in human diabetes by TNF or TNF receptor 2 agonism. *Proc Natl Acad Sci U S A.* 2008;105(36):13644–13649.

168. Qin HY, Chaturvedi P, Singh B. In vivo apoptosis of diabetogenic T cells in NOD mice by IFN-gamma/TNF-alpha. *Int Immunol.* 2004;16(12):1723–1732.

169. Hayashi T, Faustman DL. Role of defective apoptosis in type 1 diabetes and other autoimmune diseases. *Recent Prog Horm Res.* 2003;58:131–153.

170. Ramos-Casals M, Brito-Zeron P, Soto MJ, Cuadrado MJ, Khamashta MA. Autoimmune diseases induced by TNF-targeted therapies. *Best Pract Res Clin Rheumatol.* 2008;22(5):847–861.

171. van Oosten BW, et al. Increased MRI activity and immune activation in two multiple sclerosis patients treated with the monoclonal anti-tumor necrosis factor antibody cA2. *Neurology.* 1996;47(6):1531–1534.

172. Boulton JG, Bourne JT. Unstable diabetes in a patient receiving anti-TNF-alpha for rheumatoid arthritis. *Rheumatology (Oxford).* 2007;46(1):178–179.

173. Hernandez-Pando R, et al. Persistence of DNA from *Mycobacterium tuberculosis* in superficially normal lung tissue during latent infection. *Lancet.* 2000;356(9248):2133.

174. Macovei L, et al. The hidden 'mycobacteriome' of the human healthy oral cavity and upper respiratory tract. *J Oral Microbiol.* 2015;7:26094.

175. Schulz O, Pabst O. Antigen sampling in the small intestine. *Trends Immunol.* 2013;34(4):155–161.

176. Pontiroli A, et al. Prospecting environmental mycobacteria: combined molecular approaches reveal unprecedented diversity. *PLoS One.* 2013;8(7):e68648.

177. Kaevska M, Lvoncik S, Slana I, Kulich P, Kralik P. Microscopy, culture, and quantitative real-time PCR examination confirm internalization of mycobacteria in plants. *Appl Environ Microbiol.* 2014;80(13):3888–3894.

178. Fine PE, et al. Environmental mycobacteria in northern Malawi: implications for the epidemiology of tuberculosis and leprosy. *Epidemiol Infect.* 2001;126(3):379–387.

179. Sangari FJ, Parker A, Bermudez LE. *Mycobacterium avium* interaction with macrophages and intestinal epithelial cells. *Front Biosci.* 1999;4:D582–588.

180. Gomez-Smith CK, LaPara TM, Hozalski RM. Sulfate reducing Bacteria and mycobacteria dominate the biofilm communities in a Chloraminated drinking water distribution system. *Environ Sci Technol.* 2015;49(14):8432–8440.

181. Revetta RP, Gomez-Alvarez V, Gerke TL, Santo Domingo JW, Ashbolt NJ. Changes in bacterial composition of biofilm in a metropolitan drinking water distribution system. *J Appl Microbiol.* 2016;121(1):294–305.

182. Hershkovitz I, et al. Detection and molecular characterization of 9000-year-old *Mycobacterium tuberculosis* from a Neolithic settlement in the eastern Mediterranean. *PLoS One.* 2008;3(10):e3426.

183. Williams AC, Dunbar RI. Big brains, meat, tuberculosis and the nicotinamide switches: co-evolutionary relationships with modern repercussions on longevity and disease? *Med Hypotheses*. 2014;83(1):79–87.

184. Barrios-Payan J, et al. Extrapulmonary location of *Mycobacterium tuberculosis* DNA during latent infection. *J Infect Dis*. 2012;206(8):1194–1205.

185. Gomez de Aguero M, et al. The maternal microbiota drives early postnatal innate immune development. *Science*. 2016;351(6279):1296–1302.

186. Lowry CA, et al. The microbiota, immunoregulation, and mental health: implications for public health. *Curr Environ Health Rep*. 2016;3(3):270–286.

187. Parkash O. T regulatory cells and BCG as a vaccine against tuberculosis: an overview. *World J Vac*. 2015;5:96–105.

188. Henao-Tamayo MI, et al. Effect of Bacillus Calmette-Guerin vaccination on $CD4^{+-}$ $Foxp3^{+}$ T cells during acquired immune response to *Mycobacterium tuberculosis* infection. *J Leukoc Biol*. 2016;99(4):605–617.

189. Coulombe F, et al. Increased NOD2-mediated recognition of N-glycolyl muramyl dipeptide. *J Exp Med*. 2009;206(8):1709–1716.

190. Netea MG, van Crevel R. BCG-induced protection: effects on innate immune memory. *Semin Immunol*. 2014;26(6):512–517.

191. Kleinnijenhuis J, van Crevel R, Netea MG. Trained immunity: consequences for the heterologous effects of BCG vaccination. *Trans R Soc Trop Med Hyg*. 2015;109(1): 29–35.

192. Moreau M, et al. Inoculation of Bacillus Calmette-Guerin to mice induces an acute episode of sickness behavior followed by chronic depressive-like behavior. *Brain Behav Immun*. 2008;22(7):1087–1095.

193. O'Connor JC, et al. Induction of IDO by Bacille Calmette-Guerin is responsible for development of murine depressive-like behavior. *J Immunol*. 2009;182(5):3202–3212.

194. Allen HF, et al. Effect of Bacillus Calmette-Guerin vaccination on new-onset type 1 diabetes. A randomized clinical study. *Diabetes Care*. 1999;22(10):1703–1707.

195. Elliott JF, Marlin KL, Couch RM. Effect of Bacille Calmette-Guerin vaccination on C-peptide secretion in children newly diagnosed with IDDM. *Diabetes Care*. 1998;21(10):1691–1693.

196. Shehadeh N, et al. Effect of adjuvant therapy on development of diabetes in mouse and man. *Lancet*. 1994;343(8899):706–707.

197. Pozzilli P. BCG vaccine in insulin-dependent diabetes mellitus. IMDIAB Group. *Lancet*. 1997;349(9064):1520–1521.

198. Faustman DL, et al. Proof-of-concept, randomized, controlled clinical trial of Bacillus Calmette-Guerin for treatment of long-term type 1 diabetes. *PLoS One*. 2012;7(8):e41756.

199. Ristori G, et al. Use of Bacille Calmette-Guerin (BCG) in multiple sclerosis. *Neurology*. 1999;53(7):1588–1589.

200. Paolillo A, et al. The effect of Bacille Calmette-Guerin on the evolution of new enhancing lesions to hypointense T1 lesions in relapsing remitting MS. *J Neurol*. 2003;250(2):247–248.

201. Ristori G, et al. Effects of Bacille Calmette-Guerin after the first demyelinating event in the CNS. *Neurology*. 2014;82(1):41–48.

202. Rook GAW. Mycobacteria, immunoregulation, and autoimmunity. In: Faustman DL, ed. *The Value of BCG and TNF in Autoimmunity*. Boston: Academic Press; 2014:1–26.

203. Karaci M, Aydin M. The effect of BCG vaccine in protection from type 1 diabetes mellitus. *J Contemp Med*. 2012;2(1):1–8.

204. von Reyn CF, et al. Prevention of tuberculosis in Bacille Calmette-Guerin-primed, HIV-infected adults boosted with an inactivated whole-cell mycobacterial vaccine. *AIDS*. 2010;24(5):675–685.

205. Stanford JL, Stanford CA, O'Brien ME, Grange JM. Successful immunotherapy with *Mycobacterium vaccae* in the treatment of adenocarcinoma of the lung. *Eur J Cancer*. 2008;44(2):224–227.

206. Zuany-Amorim C, et al. Long-term protective and antigen-specific effect of heat-killed *Mycobacterium vaccae* in a murine model of allergic pulmonary inflammation. *J Immunol*. 2002;169(3):1492.

207. Zuany-Amorim C, et al. Suppression of airway eosinophilia by killed *Mycobacterium vaccae*-induced allergen-specific regulatory T-cells. *Nat Med*. 2002;8:625–629.

208. Le Bert N, Chain BM, Rook G, Noursadeghi M. DC priming by *M. vaccae* inhibits Th2 responses in contrast to specific TLR2 priming and is associated with selective activation of the CREB pathway. *PLoS One*. 2011;6(4):e18346.

209. Rook GA, et al. Mycobacteria and other environmental organisms as immunomodulators for immunoregulatory disorders. *Springer Semin Immunopathol*. 2004;25(3–4): 237–255.

210. Su LF, Kidd BA, Han A, Kotzin JJ, Davis MM. Virus-specific CD4(+) memory-phenotype T cells are abundant in unexposed adults. *Immunity*. 2013;38(2):373–383.

CHAPTER 10

mTORC1 Links Cellular Metabolism and Immune Functions in *Mycobacterium tuberculosis* Infection and BCG Vaccination

Valentina Guerrini, Natalie Bruiners, Maria Laura Gennaro

Public Health Research Institute, New Jersey Medical School, Rutgers, The State University of New Jersey, Newark, NJ, United States

Contents

INTRODUCTION

The Bacillus Calmette-Guérin (BCG) strain is an attenuated variant of *Mycobacterium bovis,* a member of the *Mycobacterium tuberculosis* complex. Although the BCG strain was developed as a vaccine against tuberculosis,[1] its administration has shown nonspecific, beneficial effects on various diseases, ranging from bladder cancer, asthma, multiple sclerosis, insulin–dependent diabetes, and various infections.[2] Other favorable effects on a child's health are described in other chapters of this book. Although much of the literature reports on efficacy and safety studies, the underlying mechanisms of the beneficial effects of BCG administration are generally understudied.

Given the phylogenetic similarities between BCG and virulent species of the *M. tuberculosis* complex, it is possible that knowledge gaps on the

The Value of BCG and TNF in Autoimmunity
https://doi.org/10.1016/B978-0-12-814603-3.00010-0

mechanisms by which BCG helps reduce morbidity and/or severity of various diseases can be filled by utilizing knowledge developed in studies on the pathogenesis of tuberculosis, a chronic inflammatory disease caused by *M. tuberculosis*.

M. tuberculosis is an intracellular pathogen that primarily infects macrophages, key effectors of innate immune responses. Macrophage infection, which typically occurs in the lung alveoli, is followed by migration of the infected cell into the lung parenchyma. The initiation of a local inflammatory process together with the recruitment of other innate immune cells and of primed lymphocytes lead to the formation of a multicellular aggregate called the granuloma. The evolution of the granuloma toward control of infection or excess inflammation and tissue damage determines the evolution of infection toward a chronic, asymptomatic state (latent tuberculosis infection) or an active disease process (active tuberculosis). How macrophages respond to the presence of the intracellular pathogen and how they engage the adaptive immune effectors determine infection outcome.[3]

It is becoming increasingly clear that immune functions are tightly linked with cellular metabolism, and that changes in intracellular metabolic pathways alter the function of immune cells.[4] In this chapter, we review our current understanding of the effects of *M. tuberculosis* infection on aspects of macrophage central metabolism associated with macrophage function. These may help explain some of the protective effects—specific and nonspecific—exerted by BCG administration.

INTERSECTIONS BETWEEN CELLULAR METABOLISM AND IMMUNE FUNCTION

Immune cells express functions important for host protection and tissue homeostasis. When immune responses are activated and inflammation is ongoing, immune cells express various functions, depending on the nature of the external signal and cell type. For example, they can migrate from one tissue to another, modulate surface receptor expression, clonally expand, secrete copious amounts of effector molecules, and/or exert controlling effects over neighboring cells.[5] It is increasingly recognized that alterations in immune activation represent significant metabolic stresses requiring efficient reprogramming of cellular metabolism.

Cellular metabolism produces ATP to provide energy for cellular functions. The production of ATP from glucose occurs through two integrated processes. First, glucose is metabolized to pyruvate via glycolysis; then pyruvate is oxidized to CO_2 in the mitochondria by the tricarboxylic acid (TCA) cycle and oxidative phosphorylation (OXPHOS). When oxygen is limiting, cells use only anaerobic glycolysis as source of energy, which is less efficient than OXPHOS for generating ATP. Aerobic glycolysis, in which pyruvate is converted to lactate instead of entering the TCA cycle regardless of the presence of oxygen, is a phenomenon first described in cancer cells as the "Warburg effect."[6,7] This metabolic switch meets the energy supplies of rapidly proliferating cells, such as cancer cells, by allowing for faster turn-over rate of ATP via glycolysis and facilitating the uptake and incorporation of nutrients in the biomass needed for cell proliferation.[7,8] It is now recognized that aerobic glycolysis, together with changes in lipid and amino acid metabolism, also occurs in activated immune cells, and that metabolic reprogramming is key to the effective expression of immune functions.

In macrophages, the link between metabolism and immune function has been long established. Indeed the initial definition of functional subsets of macrophages is based on amino acid metabolism.[9] When macrophages are activated with lipopolysaccharide (LPS) and the cytokine IFNγ, arginine is converted into nitric oxide (NO) via inducible NO synthase (iNOS) activity,[9–11] defining M1 macrophages. These macrophages are characterized by enhanced proinflammatory cytokine production and antimicrobial functions such as phagocytosis.[12] In contrast, M2 macrophages, activated by the cytokine IL-4, metabolize arginine by arginase-1.[13–15] These macrophages likely include multiple functional subsets expressing antiinflammatory and tissue repair functions.[12] Broader metabolic differences exist among macrophage subsets. M1 macrophages exhibit enhanced glycolysis and reduced OXPHOS, as also seen with activated dendritic cells,[16] whereas OXPHOS is induced in M2 macrophages.[4,17] In addition to glycolysis, carbon flux in M1 macrophages is also rerouted through the pentose phosphate pathway (PPP),[18] which is required for the production of nucleotide and amino acid precursors, and favors fatty acid biosynthesis. Furthermore, the TCA cycle is disrupted in two points in proinflammatory macrophages, leading to accumulation of two intermediate metabolites, citrate and succinate.[4,19] Succinate accumulation has a direct impact on proinflammatory cytokine production, particularly IL-1β,[20] whereas citrate is used to generate fatty acids for membrane biogenesis and prostaglandin production, and antimicrobial compounds.[4,21,22] Fatty acid biosynthesis affects cell membrane organization and composition, with critical effects on inflammatory signaling[23] In contrast, an intact TCA cycle, increased fatty acid oxidation, and enhanced OXPHOS are characteristic of the M2 macrophage phenotype.[24–26]

Recent reports reveal additional complexities. For example, the M2 phenotype also requires enhanced glucose utilization,[27] and the M1 and M2 macrophage activation programs may depend on relative fluxes through PPP.[28] In conclusion, although detailed mechanisms still need elucidating, very little doubt exists that macrophage activation programs are very tightly linked to metabolic regulation.

AEROBIC GLYCOLYSIS IS ACTIVATED IN IMMUNE CELLS VIA THE AKT-mTORC1-HIF PATHWAY

Aerobic glycolysis in activated macrophages and dendritic cells occurs upon ligand binding of various toll-like receptors (TLR), including TLR2,[29,30] TLR3,[29] TLR4,[29–31] TLR7/8[29] and TLR9.[29,30] It has also been reported in macrophages infected with *Bordetella pertussis*,[20] *M. tuberculosis*,[32] and *Salmonella typhimurium*.[33] The shift of immune cell metabolism toward aerobic glycolysis involves increased expression of facilitators of glucose transport, which enable uptake of glucose in an environment in which nutrient availability is reduced by inflammation. Although glucose is essential for immune activation, effector cells adapt quickly and efficiently to low glucose levels by increasing the uptake of glutamine and inducing glutaminolysis to generate substrates for the TCA cycle.[34] The metabolic switch to aerobic glycolysis is promoted by the transcription factor HIF-1α, which binds to hypoxia response elements in target genes such as glucose transport GLUT1 and glycolytic enzymes.[35–37] HIF-1α increases the abundance of lactate dehydrogenase (LDH), which catalyzes lactate production from pyruvate, thereby limiting the production of acetyl-CoA for the TCA cycle. HIF-1α also induces the levels of pyruvate dehydrogenase kinase,[38,39] leading to the inhibition of pyruvate dehydrogenase, which converts pyruvate to acetyl-CoA. The centrality of HIF-1α in glycolytic energy production and ultimately inflammation was demonstrated by decreased cellular pools of ATP and impaired bacterial killing in HIF-1α deficient macrophages.[40] Moreover, inhibition of glycolysis in LPS-activated macrophages with 2-deoxyglucose (2DG) decreases the inflammatory response, whereas inhibitors of OXPHOS have no effect, consistent with the fact that mitochondrial respiration is already switched off.[41] In LPS-induced macrophages, 2DG also reduces the production of the proinflammatory cytokine IL-1β and inhibits HIF-1α activation.[42] In HIF-1α deficient macrophages, expression of iNOS after stimulation with IFNγ is also reduced,[42] and these cells lose the ability to suppress bacterial growth.[43]

Many studies have implicated two serine/threonine protein kinases, protein kinase B (Akt) and mammalian target of rapamycin complex 1 (mTORC1), in the regulation of HIF-1α and transcription of glycolytic and glucose transport enzymes. Both protein kinases are active in the presence of excess nutrients, active proliferating cells, and metabolically demanding conditions, for example, after TLR stimulation.[44] mTORC1 controls the expression of HIF-1α by promoting the translation of mRNAs containing 5′-terminal oligopyrimidine (5′-TOP) signals, which are present in the HIF-1α mRNA.[45] Raptor, one of the components of mTORC1, interacts with HIF-1α via the signaling motif located in HIF-1α mRNA, which promotes HIF-1α activity.[46] By increasing the expression of HIF-1α, mTORC1 helps cells meet their high metabolic demand by increasing the expression of glycolytic genes and inflammatory genes.[47] Also the activation of the phosphatidylinositol 3-kinase (PI3K)/Akt pathway regulates multiple steps involved in glycolysis. The underlying mechanisms include (i) activation of mTORC1, directly (through the phosphorylation of the PRAS40 subunit) and indirectly (by inactivating TSC2, which suppresses the activity of the Rheb GTPase, an activator of mTORC1);[48,49] (ii) induction of the Glut1 gene (glucose uptake) and of hexokinase activity,[50] which converts glucose to glucose-6-phosphate in the first step of glycolysis; and (iii) activation of ATP citrate lyase to enhance the conversion of citrate to acetyl-CoA[51] needed to initiate fatty acid biosynthesis.

INTRACELLULAR PATHOGENS AND mTORC1

Several intracellular pathogens manipulate the mTORC1 pathway in innate immune cells by directly targeting mTORC1 or modulating the upstream or downstream pathways.[52] Various consequences have been described. For example, some viruses, such as the hepatitis C virus, benefit from mTORC1 activation to complete their replication cycle.[53] In the case of intracellular bacteria, at least two types of scenarios have been reported, both related to mTORC1-mediated inhibition of autophagy, a mechanism of cytoplasmic quality and quantity control in eukaryotic cells.[54] Most typically, immune cells utilize autophagy to target intracellular pathogens to lysosomes, thereby restricting their replication and survival.[55] Consequently, intracellular bacteria such as *M. tuberculosis* and *S. typhimurium* benefit from mTORC1-mediated block of autophagy to escape immune elimination.[56,57] However, other intracellular pathogens use autophagy to their own advantage: blocking mTORC1 activity leads to induction of autophagy, degradation of cytosolic components, and increased nutrient availability for the pathogen.[58] One such example is *Francisella tularensis*.[59] Some other pathogens, such *Yersinia pseudotuberculosis* and *Coxiella* spp., hijack the autophagy pathway and replicate inside nonacidified autophagosomes.[60,61]

M. tuberculosis positively regulates the mTORC1 pathway in immune cells, as first reported in 2012[62] and further demonstrated in later studies.[63] In the following, we summarize two effects of *M. tuberculosis*-induced activation of mTORC1 in host immune cells: (i) host cell metabolic reprogramming toward aerobic glycolysis (the Warburg effect) and (ii) block of autophagy.

M. TUBERCULOSIS-INDUCED METABOLIC REMODELING OF HOST IMMUNE CELLS

A metabolic shift to aerobic glycolysis has been shown during *M. tuberculosis* infection.[64] In a murine model of tuberculosis, transcriptomic analyses of infected lungs revealed gene expression changes consistent with the Warburg effect.[65] These included increased expression of genes encoding glucose transporters and glycolytic enzymes, and downregulation of genes involved in the TCA cycle and OXPHOS. In addition, immunohistochemistry showed increased abundance of glycolytic enzymes in macrophages and T cells in lung granulomas from the same animals.[65] Consistent with these observations, accumulation of lactate, the product of glycolysis, was observed in *M. tuberculosis*-infected mouse lungs by metabolomics.[66] Gene expression changes consistent with the Warburg effect were also reported in tuberculous rabbits[67] and in lung granulomas of individuals with active tuberculosis.[68]

Only a few mechanistic and functional studies have been performed on aerobic glycolysis in immune cells during *M. tuberculosis* infection. Induction of aerobic glycolysis has been reported with several types of macrophages infected with *M. tuberculosis* in vitro.[63,69] Using human peripheral blood mononuclear cells (PBMC), it has been shown that the *M. tuberculosis*-induced shift toward aerobic glycolysis occurs in a TLR2-dependent and NOD2-independent manner.[63] The same study also showed that this metabolic reprogramming is mediated in part through activation of Akt-mTORC1 pathway in *M. tuberculosis*-infected human and mouse macrophages.[63] Moreover, because HIF-1α expression is increased in tuberculous lesions in mouse lungs,[65] it has been proposed that HIF-1α is a key regulator of the metabolic reprogramming occurring in immune cells during *M. tuberculosis* infection.[63,65]

The host immune cell metabolic rewiring induced by *M. tuberculosis* infection has been associated with a proinflammatory macrophage phenotype and with infection outcome.[63,64,69] Inhibition of the shift from OXPHOS to aerobic glycolysis by 2-deoxyglucose resulted in decreased levels of the proinflammatory cytokine IL-1β, required for host resistance to *M. tuberculosis*,[70] and increased levels of the antiinflammatory cytokine IL-10 in *M. tuberculosis*-infected macrophages.[69] Consistent with these data, expression of genes coding for glycolysis or TCA cycle enzymes in PBMC differed among healthy donors, latently infected individuals, and active tuberculosis patients.[63]

Further insight derives from studies comparing infection with different *M. tuberculosis* strains. Transcriptomic analysis of murine bone marrow-derived macrophages (BMDM) infected with the CDC1551 and HN878 strains of *M. tuberculosis* revealed that, although a similar set of Warburg effect-associated genes was induced by both strains, macrophages infected with the CDC1551 strain were characterized by high glycolytic flux and high expression of inflammatory and antimicrobial effector molecules, yet macrophages infected with the HN878 strain had elevated glucose uptake and lower glycolytic flux.[71] Because these strains induce differential immune responses in BMDM,[71] a link may exist between host metabolic state and immune response. Studies in zebrafish infected with *Mycobacterium marinum* (a fish model of tuberculosis) also demonstrated a role for HIF-1α in antimycobacterial responses, leading to the proposal of stabilization of HIF-1α as potential target for therapeutic intervention against tuberculosis.[72]

M. TUBERCULOSIS AND AUTOPHAGY

Autophagy maintains cellular homeostasis by delivering cytosolic components to lysosomes for degradation in response to environmental changes. For example, during nutrient deprivation, autophagy is activated to degrade cytosolic components and generate sufficient nutrients to support cell viability. In addition to its housekeeping functions, autophagy is utilized by the cells to sense, sequester, and destroy intracellular microorganisms, and is a component of both innate and adaptive immunity.[73] The autophagic process is induced in response to immunological modulators, such as pattern recognition receptor ligands and cytokines, and pharmacological compounds.[74,75] As previously mentioned, a major regulator of autophagy is mTORC1,[76] which links regulation of carbon metabolism and autophagy.[77] mTORC1 negatively regulates autophagy by phosphorylating UNC-51-like kinase

1 (ULK1) and inhibiting its activity.[78] The AMP-activated protein kinase (AMPK), a sensor of nutrient deprivation,[79] positively regulates autophagy by directly inhibiting mTORC1 and by activating ULK1 through phosphorylation at a different amino acid residue.[80]

Autophagy has an important role during *M. tuberculosis* infection, as its induction by physiological or pharmacological stimuli[81,82] positively regulates several protective immune functions. These include: (i) maturation and acidification of *M. tuberculosis*-containing phagosomes, which counter the *M. tuberculosis*-mediated block of phagosome-lysosome fusion;[83–86] (ii) release of antigenic fragments from lysosome-degraded bacteria and antigen presentation;[87] and (iii) control of inflammatory response to avoid excess inflammation[88,89] and promote bacterial clearance.[90] The protective effects of autophagy in tuberculosis are further supported by the observation that transgenic autophagy-defective mice infected with *M. tuberculosis* exhibited higher bacillary burden and more severe lung pathology.[83]

Inhibition of the autophagic flux during *M. tuberculosis* infection has been described in several reports,[91–93] and some mycobacterial factors express antiautophagic activity.[94–96] Inhibition of autophagy by mycobacteria was concurrent with mTORC1 activation, suggesting the possibility that mycobacteria activate mTORC1 to block or slow down autophagy.[62] Indeed, nutrient starvation (which leads to mTORC1 inactivation) and treatment with rapamycin (a chemical inhibitor of mTORC1) reduced *M. tuberculosis* growth in macrophages.[83]

In light of the mechanisms previously described, it can be concluded that the effects of mTORC1 activity on the outcome of *M. tuberculosis* infection are complex. On one hand, mTORC1-dependent metabolic remodeling is necessary to control tuberculosis infection. On the other, mTORC1-mediated inhibition of autophagy promotes intracellular bacterial survival. Consequently, the effects of therapies targeting mTORC1 may vary. For example, several compounds targeting mTORC1 have been found to stimulate autophagy and *M. tuberculosis* killing.[97,98] Interestingly, autophagy is required for effective antibacterial activity by standard antitubercular regimen drugs.[99] However, adverse effects of mTORC1 inhibition have also been observed. For example, treatment with mTORC1 inhibitors of macrophages singly or doubly infected with HIV and *M. tuberculosis* was shown to accelerate mycobacterial replication.[100] Thus, further investigation is needed to fully understand the role of mTORC1 during *M. tuberculosis* infection, and antituberculosis therapeutic regimens targeting the mTORC1 pathway will have to be carefully evaluated.

TRAINED IMMUNITY, AEROBIC GLYCOLYSIS, AND BCG

The metabolic reprogramming occurring in tuberculous macrophages previously described and the nonspecific beneficial effects afforded by BCG administration are likely linked through a mechanism referred to as "trained immunity."[101] Trained immunity refers to the adaptive changes induced in innate immune cells (myeloid cells and natural killer cells) in response to a stimulus, for example, exposure to β-glucan from fungi.[102,103] Given the very nature of innate immune functions, the increased responsiveness to secondary stimuli that characterizes trained immunity is not antigen/pathogen-specific. At least two mechanisms have been associated with trained immunity. One is epigenetic reprogramming. Profiling of histone marks and DNAse I cleavage sensitivity demonstrated epigenetic changes associated with β-glucan training of myeloid cells.[104] The second is aerobic glycolysis. β-Glucan-trained monocytes exhibited elevated aerobic glycolysis; this metabolic shift required dectin 1 (a surface receptor for β-glucan) and the Akt-mTORC1-HIF-1α signaling pathway.[103] Furthermore, mice lacking myeloid-specific HIF-1α were unable to express trained immunity in response to sepsis.[103] Epigenetic and metabolic mechanisms are tightly intertwined. For example, accumulation of fumarate, a TCA cycle metabolite, induces monocyte epigenetic reprogramming by inhibiting KDM5 histone demethylases.[105] Moreover, β-glucan-training of myeloid cells is associated with histone modification and upregulation of glycolysis genes.[103,104] Furthermore, histone acetylation of glycolytic genes, which promotes glycolysis, requires the cellular functions involved in transport of citrate, another TCA cycle intermediate, to the cytosol.[106] Glutamine metabolism is also linked to expression of trained immunity in multiple ways, for example, by replenishing TCA cycle intermediates.[106]

Although much of the trained immunity experimentation has utilized β-glucan (e.g., 102–104), initial studies support the idea that trained immunity may also mediate the nonspecific protective effects against infections afforded by live vaccines, such as BCG and measles.[107,108] Vaccination of healthy volunteers with BCG induced epigenetic changes in myeloid cells and cytokine production by monocytes challenged ex vivo with unrelated pathogens.[109] In mice, the BCG-protective effects against heterologous challenge were independent of functional B- and T-cells,[109] confirming the innate immune nature of the phenomenon. Moreover, BCG induction of trained immunity in human and murine monocytes was accompanied by increased glycolysis and glutamine metabolism, and required activation of the Akt-mTORC1 pathway.[110] Furthermore, histone marks of gene activation were found at the promoters of mTOR and key glycolytic genes,[110] linking metabolic and epigenetic changes. A summary of the cellular events associated with BCG-induced trained immunity is shown in Fig. 10.1. Initial studies on patients' cohorts corroborate the mechanistic findings. For example, the presence of a cytokine/chemokine biomarker signature of trained immunity has been recently proposed in BCG-vaccinated neonates,[111] which may help explain the reported protection against all-cause mortality afforded by BCG vaccination at birth.[112,113]

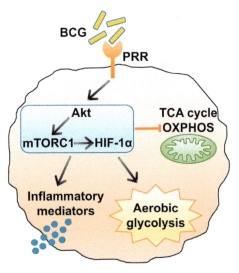

Fig. 10.1 Metabolic basis of BCG-induced trained immunity in macrophages. Naïve macrophages during aerobic conditions use tricarboxylic acid (TCA) cycle and oxidative phosphorylation (OXPHOS) to generate adenosine triphosphate (ATP) as an energy source. When BCG components bind to macrophage pattern recognition receptors (PRR), the pathway including protein kinase B (Akt), mammalian target of rapamycin complex 1 (mTORC1), and hypoxia-inducible factor 1 (HIF-1) is activated. As a result, glucose metabolism shifts from TCA cycle/OXPHOS to aerobic glycolysis. The resulting macrophage is "trained," because the activated metabolic state prepares the cell to respond to secondary stimuli. The BCG-trained macrophage exhibits high glucose consumption, high lactate production, high ratio of nicotinamide adenine dinucleotide (NAD+) to its reduced form (NADH), and increased production of mediators of inflammation. These characteristics make the immune functions of the trained macrophage more effective and result in protective responses to unrelated infectious and noninfectious stimuli.

CONCLUSIONS

The beneficial effects of the administration of the BCG vaccine strain vastly surpass those associated with protection from complications of neonatal tuberculosis. These effects are nonspecific, as they apply to diseases caused by nonrelated infectious agents or of noninfectious nature. Trained immunity, a means of the innate immune system to retain memory, is associated with deeply intertwined epigenetic and metabolic changes in innate immune cells. One such metabolic change is the shift to aerobic glycolysis, which is regulated by the Akt-mTORC1-HIF-1α pathway. Similar changes also occur during macrophage infection with virulent *M. tuberculosis*, a bacterial species closely related to the BCG strain. Thus mechanistic studies of macrophage metabolic responses to tuberculosis and of myeloid cell changes associated with the nonspecific beneficial effects of BCG may complement each other, contribute new insight in phenomena occurring during host exposure to mycobacteria, and lead to new immunotherapies.

REFERENCES

1. Fletcher HA. Sleeping beauty and the story of the Bacille Calmette-Guerin vaccine. *MBio*. 2016;7(4):e01370-16.
2. Faustman DL. *The Value of BCG and TNF in Autoimmunity*. 1st ed. Cambridge: Elsevier Science and Technology Books; 2014.
3. Flynn JL, Chan J, Lin PL. Macrophages and control of granulomatous inflammation in tuberculosis. *Mucosal Immunol*. 2011;4:271–278.
4. O'Neill LA, Kishton RJ, Rathmell J. A guide to immunometabolism for immunologists. *Nat Rev Immunol*. 2016;16:553–565.
5. Buck MD, Sowell RT, Kaech SM, Pearce EL. Metabolic instruction of immunity. *Cell*. 2017;169:570–586.
6. Warburg O. On the origin of cancer cells. *Science*. 1956;123:309–314.
7. Vander Heiden MG, Cantley LC, Thompson CB. Understanding the Warburg effect: the metabolic requirements of cell proliferation. *Science*. 2009;324:1029–1033.
8. Alfarouk KO, Verduzco D, Rauch C, et al. Glycolysis, tumor metabolism, cancer growth and dissemination. A new pH-based etiopathogenic perspective and therapeutic approach to an old cancer question. *Oncoscience*. 2014;1:777–802.
9. Munder M, Eichmann K, Modolell M. Alternative metabolic states in murine macrophages reflected by the nitric oxide synthase/arginase balance: competitive regulation by CD4+ T cells correlates with Th1/Th2 phenotype. *J Immunol*. 1998;160:5347–5354.
10. Murray PJ, Allen JE, Biswas SK, et al. Macrophage activation and polarization: nomenclature and experimental guidelines. *Immunity*. 2014;41:14–20.
11. Ajayi AA, Matsuda K, Schror K, Masuda A, Mathur R, Halushka PV. Androgen regulation of thromboxane A2 receptors. *Adv Prostaglandin Thromboxane Leukot Res*. 1995;23:251–253.
12. Martinez FO, Helming L, Gordon S. Alternative activation of macrophages: an immunologic functional perspective. *Annu Rev Immunol*. 2009;27:451–483.

13. Van den Bossche J, Lamers WH, Koehler ES, et al. Pivotal advance: arginase-1-independent polyamine production stimulates the expression of IL-4-induced alternatively activated macrophage markers while inhibiting LPS-induced expression of inflammatory genes. *J Leukoc Biol.* 2012;91:685–699.

14. Corraliza IM, Soler G, Eichmann K, Modolell M. Arginase induction by suppressors of nitric oxide synthesis (IL-4, IL-10 and PGE2) in murine bone-marrow-derived macrophages. *Biochem Biophys Res Commun.* 1995;206:667–673.

15. Modolell M, Corraliza IM, Link F, Soler G, Eichmann K. Reciprocal regulation of the nitric oxide synthase/arginase balance in mouse bone marrow-derived macrophages by TH1 and TH2 cytokines. *Eur J Immunol.* 1995;25:1101–1104.

16. O'Neill LA. Glycolytic reprogramming by TLRs in dendritic cells. *Nat Immunol.* 2014;15:314–315.

17. Pearce EL, Pearce EJ. Metabolic pathways in immune cell activation and quiescence. *Immunity.* 2013;38:633–643.

18. Nagy C, Haschemi A. Time and demand are two critical dimensions of Immunometabolism: the process of macrophage activation and the pentose phosphate pathway. *Front Immunol.* 2015;6:164.

19. O'Neill LA. A broken Krebs cycle in macrophages. *Immunity.* 2015;42:393–394.

20. Tannahill GM, Curtis AM, Adamik J, et al. Succinate is an inflammatory signal that induces IL-1beta through HIF-1alpha. *Nature.* 2013;496:238–242.

21. Infantino V, Iacobazzi V, Palmieri F, Menga A. ATP-citrate lyase is essential for macrophage inflammatory response. *Biochem Biophys Res Commun.* 2013;440:105–111.

22. Infantino V, Convertini P, Cucci L, et al. The mitochondrial citrate carrier: a new player in inflammation. *Biochem J.* 2011;438:433–436.

23. Wei X, Song H, Yin L, et al. Fatty acid synthesis configures the plasma membrane for inflammation in diabetes. *Nature.* 2016;539:294–298.

24. Odegaard JI, Chawla A. Alternative macrophage activation and metabolism. *Annu Rev Pathol.* 2011;6:275–297.

25. Van den Bossche J, Baardman J, de Winther MP. Metabolic characterization of polarized M1 and M2 bone marrow-derived macrophages using real-time extracellular flux analysis. *J Vis Exp.* 2015; https://doi.org/10.3791/53424.

26. Huang SC, Everts B, Ivanova Y, et al. Cell-intrinsic lysosomal lipolysis is essential for alternative activation of macrophages. *Nat Immunol.* 2014;15:846–855.

27. Huang SC, Smith AM, Everts B, et al. Metabolic reprogramming mediated by the mTORC2-IRF4 signaling axis is essential for macrophage alternative activation. *Immunity.* 2016;45:817–830.

28. Haschemi A, Kosma P, Gille L, et al. The sedoheptulose kinase CARKL directs macrophage polarization through control of glucose metabolism. *Cell Metab.* 2012;15:813–826.

29. Everts B, Amiel E, Huang SC, et al. TLR-driven early glycolytic reprogramming via the kinases TBK1-IKKvarepsilon supports the anabolic demands of dendritic cell activation. *Nat Immunol.* 2014;15:323–332.

30. Krawczyk CM, Holowka T, Sun J, et al. Toll-like receptor-induced changes in glycolytic metabolism regulate dendritic cell activation. *Blood.* 2010;115:4742–4749.

31. Everts B, Amiel E, van der Windt GJ, et al. Commitment to glycolysis sustains survival of NO-producing inflammatory dendritic cells. *Blood.* 2012;120:1422–1431.

32. Mehrotra P, Jamwal SV, Saquib N, et al. Pathogenicity of Mycobacterium tuberculosis is expressed by regulating metabolic thresholds of the host macrophage. *PLoS Pathog.* 2014;10:e1004265.

33. Palsson-McDermott EM, Curtis AM, Goel G, et al. Pyruvate kinase M2 regulates Hif-1alpha activity and IL-1beta induction and is a critical determinant of the Warburg effect in LPS-activated macrophages. *Cell Metab.* 2015;21:65–80.

34. Jha AK, Huang SC, Sergushichev A, et al. Network integration of parallel metabolic and transcriptional data reveals metabolic modules that regulate macrophage polarization. *Immunity.* 2015;42:419–430.

35. Semenza GL, Nejfelt MK, Chi SM, Antonarakis SE. Hypoxia-inducible nuclear factors bind to an enhancer element located 3′ to the human erythropoietin gene. *Proc Natl Acad Sci USA.* 1991;88:5680–5684.

36. Mole DR, Blancher C, Copley RR, et al. Genome-wide association of hypoxia-inducible factor (HIF)-1alpha and HIF-2alpha DNA binding with expression profiling of hypoxia-inducible transcripts. *J Biol Chem.* 2009;284:16767–16775.

37. Chen C, Pore N, Behrooz A, Ismail-Beigi F, Maity A. Regulation of glut1 mRNA by hypoxia-inducible factor-1. Interaction between H-ras and hypoxia. *J Biol Chem.* 2001;276:9519–9525.

38. Kim JW, Tchernyshyov I, Semenza GL, Dang CV. HIF-1-mediated expression of pyruvate dehydrogenase kinase: a metabolic switch required for cellular adaptation to hypoxia. *Cell Metab.* 2006;3:177–185.

39. Papandreou I, Cairns RA, Fontana L, Lim AL, Denko NC. HIF-1 mediates adaptation to hypoxia by actively downregulating mitochondrial oxygen consumption. *Cell Metab.* 2006;3:187–197.

40. Cramer T, Yamanishi Y, Clausen BE, et al. HIF-1alpha is essential for myeloid cell-mediated inflammation. *Cell.* 2003;112:645–657.

41. Kellett DN. 2-Deoxyglucose and inflammation. *J Pharm Pharmacol.* 1966;18:199–200.

42. Takeda N, O'Dea EL, Doedens A, et al. Differential activation and antagonistic function of HIF-1alpha isoforms in macrophages are essential for NO homeostasis. *Genes Dev.* 2010;24:491–501.

43. Peyssonnaux C, Datta V, Cramer T, et al. HIF-1alpha expression regulates the bactericidal capacity of phagocytes. *J Clin Invest.* 2005;115:1806–1815.

44. Byles V, Covarrubias AJ, Ben-Sahra I, et al. The TSC-mTOR pathway regulates macrophage polarization. *Nat Commun.* 2013;4:2834.

45. Huo Y, Iadevaia V, Yao Z, et al. Stable isotope-labelling analysis of the impact of inhibition of the mammalian target of rapamycin on protein synthesis. *Biochem J.* 2012;444:141–151.

46. Land SC, Tee AR. Hypoxia-inducible factor 1alpha is regulated by the mammalian target of rapamycin (mTOR) via an mTOR signaling motif. *J Biol Chem.* 2007;282:20534–20543.

47. Palazon A, Goldrath AW, Nizet V, Johnson RS. HIF transcription factors, inflammation, and immunity. *Immunity.* 2014;41:518–528.

48. Huang J, Manning BD. A complex interplay between Akt, TSC2 and the two mTOR complexes. *Biochem Soc Trans.* 2009;37:217–222.

49. Memmott RM, Dennis PA. Akt-dependent and -independent mechanisms of mTOR regulation in cancer. *Cell Signal.* 2009;21:656–664.

50. Makinoshima H, Takita M, Saruwatari K, et al. Signaling through the phosphatidylinositol 3-kinase (PI3K)/mammalian target of rapamycin (mTOR) axis is responsible for aerobic glycolysis mediated by glucose transporter in epidermal growth factor receptor (EGFR)-mutated lung adenocarcinoma. *J Biol Chem.* 2015;290:17495–17504.

51. Hanai J, Doro N, Sasaki AT, et al. Inhibition of lung cancer growth: ATP citrate lyase knockdown and statin treatment leads to dual blockade of mitogen-activated protein kinase (MAPK) and phosphatidylinositol-3-kinase (PI3K)/AKT pathways. *J Cell Physiol.* 2012;227:1709–1720.

52. Brunton J, Steele S, Ziehr B, Moorman N, Kawula T. Feeding uninvited guests: mTOR and AMPK set the table for intracellular pathogens. *PLoS Pathog.* 2013;9:e1003552.

53. Stohr S, Costa R, Sandmann L, et al. Host cell mTORC1 is required for HCV RNA replication. *Gut.* 2016;65:2017–2028.

54. Murrow L, Debnath J. Autophagy as a stress-response and quality-control mechanism: implications for cell injury and human disease. *Annu Rev Pathol*. 2013;8:105–137.
55. Jo EK, Yuk JM, Shin DM, Sasakawa C. Roles of autophagy in elimination of intracellular bacterial pathogens. *Front Immunol*. 2013;4:97.
56. Kimmey JM, Stallings CL. Bacterial pathogens versus autophagy: implications for therapeutic interventions. *Trends Mol Med*. 2016;22:1060–1076.
57. Owen KA, Meyer CB, Bouton AH, Casanova JE. Activation of focal adhesion kinase by Salmonella suppresses autophagy via an Akt/mTOR signaling pathway and promotes bacterial survival in macrophages. *PLoS Pathog*. 2014;10:e1004159.
58. Steele S, Brunton J, Kawula T. The role of autophagy in intracellular pathogen nutrient acquisition. *Front Cell Infect Microbiol*. 2015;5:51.
59. Steele S, Brunton J, Ziehr B, Taft-Benz S, Moorman N, Kawula T. Francisella tularensis harvests nutrients derived via ATG5-independent autophagy to support intracellular growth. *PLoS Pathog*. 2013;9:e1003562.
60. Moreau K, Lacas-Gervais S, Fujita N, et al. Autophagosomes can support Yersinia pseudotuberculosis replication in macrophages. *Cell Microbiol*. 2010;12:1108–1123.
61. Gutierrez MG, Vazquez CL, Munafo DB, et al. Autophagy induction favours the generation and maturation of the Coxiella-replicative vacuoles. *Cell Microbiol*. 2005;7:981–993.
62. Zullo AJ, Lee S. Mycobacterial induction of autophagy varies by species and occurs independently of mammalian target of rapamycin inhibition. *J Biol Chem*. 2012;287:12668–12678.
63. Lachmandas E, Beigier-Bompadre M, Cheng SC, et al. Rewiring cellular metabolism via the AKT/mTOR pathway contributes to host defence against Mycobacterium tuberculosis in human and murine cells. *Eur J Immunol*. 2016;46:2574–2586.
64. Shi L, Eugenin EA, Subbian S. Immunometabolism in tuberculosis. *Front Immunol*. 2016;7:150.
65. Shi L, Salamon H, Eugenin EA, Pine R, Cooper A, Gennaro ML. Infection with Mycobacterium tuberculosis induces the Warburg effect in mouse lungs. *Sci Rep*. 2015;5:18176.
66. Shin JH, Yang JY, Jeon BY, et al. ^{1}H NMR-based metabolomic profiling in mice infected with Mycobacterium tuberculosis. *J Proteome Res*. 2011;10:2238–2247.
67. Subbian S, Tsenova L, Yang G, et al. Chronic pulmonary cavitary tuberculosis in rabbits: a failed host immune response. *Open Biol*. 2011;1:110016.
68. Subbian S, Tsenova L, Kim MJ, et al. Lesion-specific immune response in granulomas of patients with pulmonary tuberculosis: a pilot study. *PLoS One*. 2015;10:e0132249.
69. Gleeson LE, Sheedy FJ, Palsson-McDermott EM, et al. Cutting edge: Mycobacterium tuberculosis induces aerobic glycolysis in human alveolar macrophages that is required for control of intracellular bacillary replication. *J Immunol*. 2016;196:2444–2449.
70. Mayer-Barber KD, Barber DL, Shenderov K, et al. Caspase-1 independent IL-1beta production is critical for host resistance to mycobacterium tuberculosis and does not require TLR signaling in vivo. *J Immunol*. 2010;184:3326–3330.
71. Koo MS, Subbian S, Kaplan G. Strain specific transcriptional response in Mycobacterium tuberculosis infected macrophages. *Cell Commun Signal*. 2012;10:2.
72. Elks PM, Brizee S, van der Vaart M, et al. Hypoxia inducible factor signaling modulates susceptibility to mycobacterial infection via a nitric oxide dependent mechanism. *PLoS Pathog*. 2013;9:e1003789.
73. Deretic V, Saitoh T, Akira S. Autophagy in infection, inflammation and immunity. *Nat Rev Immunol*. 2013;13:722–737.
74. Kroemer G, Marino G, Levine B. Autophagy and the integrated stress response. *Mol Cell*. 2010;40:280–293.
75. Morel E, Mehrpour M, Botti J, et al. Autophagy: a druggable process. *Annu Rev Pharmacol Toxicol*. 2017;57:375–398.
76. Rabanal-Ruiz Y, Otten EG, Korolchuk VI. mTORC1 as the main gateway to autophagy. *Essays Biochem*. 2017;61:565–584.

77. Dunlop EA, Tee AR. mTOR and autophagy: a dynamic relationship governed by nutrients and energy. *Semin Cell Dev Biol.* 2014;36:121–129.
78. Gallagher LE, Williamson LE, Chan EY. Advances in autophagy regulatory mechanisms. *Cells.* 2016;5(2):E24.
79. Hardie DG, Ross FA, Hawley SA. AMPK: a nutrient and energy sensor that maintains energy homeostasis. *Nat Rev Mol Cell Biol.* 2012;13:251–262.
80. Kim J, Kundu M, Viollet B, Guan KL. AMPK and mTOR regulate autophagy through direct phosphorylation of Ulk1. *Nat Cell Biol.* 2011;13:132–141.
81. Yuk JM, Shin DM, Lee HM, et al. Vitamin D3 induces autophagy in human monocytes/macrophages via cathelicidin. *Cell Host Microbe.* 2009;6:231–243.
82. Juarez E, Carranza C, Sanchez G, et al. Loperamide restricts intracellular growth of Mycobacterium tuberculosis in lung macrophages. *Am J Respir Cell Mol Biol.* 2016;55:837–847.
83. Gutierrez MG, Master SS, Singh SB, Taylor GA, Colombo MI, Deretic V. Autophagy is a defense mechanism inhibiting BCG and Mycobacterium tuberculosis survival in infected macrophages. *Cell.* 2004;119:753–766.
84. Harris J, De Haro SA, Master SS, et al. T helper 2 cytokines inhibit autophagic control of intracellular Mycobacterium tuberculosis. *Immunity.* 2007;27:505–517.
85. Singh SB, Davis AS, Taylor GA, Deretic V. Human IRGM induces autophagy to eliminate intracellular mycobacteria. *Science.* 2006;313:1438–1441.
86. Fabri M, Stenger S, Shin DM, et al. Vitamin D is required for IFN-gamma-mediated antimicrobial activity of human macrophages. *Sci Transl Med.* 2011;3:104ra102.
87. Munz C. Autophagy proteins in antigen processing for presentation on MHC molecules. *Immunol Rev.* 2016;272:17–27.
88. Levine B, Mizushima N, Virgin HW. Autophagy in immunity and inflammation. *Nature.* 2011;469:323–335.
89. Zhong Z, Sanchez-Lopez E, Karin M. Autophagy, inflammation, and immunity: a troika governing cancer and its treatment. *Cell.* 2016;166:288–298.
90. Bradfute SB, Castillo EF, Arko-Mensah J, et al. Autophagy as an immune effector against tuberculosis. *Curr Opin Microbiol.* 2013;16:355–365.
91. Chandra P, Ghanwat S, Matta SK, et al. Mycobacterium tuberculosis inhibits RAB7 recruitment to selectively modulate autophagy flux in macrophages. *Sci Rep.* 2015;5:16320.
92. Kathania M, Raje CI, Raje M, Dutta RK, Majumdar S. Bfl-1/A1 acts as a negative regulator of autophagy in mycobacteria infected macrophages. *Int J Biochem Cell Biol.* 2011;43:573–585.
93. Espert L, Beaumelle B, Vergne I. Autophagy in Mycobacterium tuberculosis and HIV infections. *Front Cell Infect Microbiol.* 2015;5:49.
94. Shui W, Petzold CJ, Redding A, et al. Organelle membrane proteomics reveals differential influence of mycobacterial lipoglycans on macrophage phagosome maturation and autophagosome accumulation. *J Proteome Res.* 2011;10:339–348.
95. Romagnoli A, Etna MP, Giacomini E, et al. ESX-1 dependent impairment of autophagic flux by Mycobacterium tuberculosis in human dendritic cells. *Autophagy.* 2012;8:1357–1370.
96. Shin DM, Jeon BY, Lee HM, et al. Mycobacterium tuberculosis eis regulates autophagy, inflammation, and cell death through redox-dependent signaling. *PLoS Pathog.* 2010;6:e1001230.
97. Zullo AJ, Jurcic Smith KL, Lee S. Mammalian target of rapamycin inhibition and mycobacterial survival are uncoupled in murine macrophages. *BMC Biochem.* 2014;15:4.
98. Lam KK, Zheng X, Forestieri R, et al. Nitazoxanide stimulates autophagy and inhibits mTORC1 signaling and intracellular proliferation of Mycobacterium tuberculosis. *PLoS Pathog.* 2012;8:e1002691.
99. Kim JJ, Lee HM, Shin DM, et al. Host cell autophagy activated by antibiotics is required for their effective antimycobacterial drug action. *Cell Host Microbe.* 2012;11:457–468.

100. Andersson AM, Andersson B, Lorell C, Raffetseder J, Larsson M, Blomgran R. Autophagy induction targeting mTORC1 enhances Mycobacterium tuberculosis replication in HIV co-infected human macrophages. *Sci Rep.* 2016;6:28171.
101. Netea MG, Quintin J, van der Meer JW. Trained immunity: a memory for innate host defense. *Cell Host Microbe.* 2011;9:355–361.
102. Quintin J, Saeed S, Martens JHA, et al. Candida albicans infection affords protection against reinfection via functional reprogramming of monocytes. *Cell Host Microbe.* 2012;12:223–232.
103. Cheng SC, Quintin J, Cramer RA, et al. mTOR- and HIF-1alpha-mediated aerobic glycolysis as metabolic basis for trained immunity. *Science.* 2014;345:1250684.
104. Saeed S, Quintin J, Kerstens HH, et al. Epigenetic programming of monocyte-to-macrophage differentiation and trained innate immunity. *Science.* 2014;345:1251086.
105. Arts RJ, Novakovic B, Ter Horst R, et al. Glutaminolysis and fumarate accumulation integrate immunometabolic and epigenetic programs in trained immunity. *Cell Metab.* 2016;24:807–819.
106. Arts RJ, Joosten LA, Netea MG. Immunometabolic circuits in trained immunity. *Semin Immunol.* 2016;28:425–430.
107. Netea MG, Joosten LA, Latz E, et al. Trained immunity: a program of innate immune memory in health and disease. *Science.* 2016;352:aaf1098.
108. Netea MG, van der Meer JW. Trained immunity: an ancient way of remembering. *Cell Host Microbe.* 2017;21:297–300.
109. Kleinnijenhuis J, Quintin J, Preijers F, et al. Bacille Calmette-Guerin induces NOD2-dependent nonspecific protection from reinfection via epigenetic reprogramming of monocytes. *Proc Natl Acad Sci USA.* 2012;109:17537–17542.
110. Arts RJ, Carvalho A, La Rocca C, et al. Immunometabolic pathways in BCG-induced trained immunity. *Cell Rep.* 2016;17:2562–2571.
111. Smith SG, Kleinnijenhuis J, Netea MG, Dockrell HM. Whole blood profiling of Bacillus Calmette-Guerin-induced trained innate immunity in infants identifies epidermal growth factor, IL-6, platelet-derived growth factor-AB/BB, and natural killer cell activation. *Front Immunol.* 2017;8:644.
112. Aaby P, Roth A, Ravn H, et al. Randomized trial of BCG vaccination at birth to low-birth-weight children: beneficial nonspecific effects in the neonatal period? *J Infect Dis.* 2011;204:245–252.
113. Goodridge HS, Ahmed SS, Curtis N, et al. Harnessing the beneficial heterologous effects of vaccination. *Nat Rev Immunol.* 2016;16:392–400.

CHAPTER 11

The Role of Maternal Priming and Boosting for the Nonspecific Effects of BCG Vaccine

C.S. Benn*,†, A. Rieckmann*,†, K.J. Jensen*, P. Aaby*,‡

*Research Center for Vitamins and Vaccines (CVIVA), Copenhagen S, Denmark
†OPEN, Institute of Clinical Research and Danish Institute of Advanced Science, University of Southern Denmark and Odense University Hospital, Odense, Denmark
‡Bandim Health Project, Indepth Network, Bissau, Guinea-Bissau

Contents

INTRODUCTION

The live BCG vaccine has been associated with substantial reductions in all-cause mortality among children in low-income countries. Based on the available evidence, BCG reduces overall mortality by at least one-third in the age groups where BCG is the most recent vaccination. This is far more than can be explained by prevention of TB.[1–3] In a high-income country such as Denmark, BCG vaccination at school age was also associated with strong mortality reductions into early adulthood.[4] Hence, like other live vaccines,[5] BCG seems to have beneficial *nonspecific effects*.

Immunological studies have now shown that BCG induces epigenetic modifications of innate immune cells, increasing their capability to respond to subsequent unrelated pathogenic challenges[6]; thus providing a plausible mechanism by which BCG could induce important long-lasting nonspecific benefits.[7,8]

It is well known that preexisting immunity alters the *specific* immune response to a vaccine. For instance, for all childhood vaccines, presence of maternally transferred antibodies at the time of the first vaccination dampens the specific antibody response to the vaccine in the offspring.[9] Furthermore, vaccines induce immunity, which increases the subsequent antibody response to "booster" doses of the same vaccine.

Hence, we asked ourselves if preexisting immunity, maternally derived or from a previous vaccine, would modify the *nonspecific effects* of vaccines. In the present chapter, we present the evidence with respect to BCG vaccine.

MATERNAL PRIMING WITH BCG

Like the live BCG vaccine, the live measles vaccine may have beneficial nonspecific effects.[5] For measles vaccine, we recently reported that the beneficial nonspecific effects on overall mortality were much stronger if the children had been measles vaccinated in the presence of maternal measles antibodies than if they had been measles vaccinated in the absence of maternal antibodies.[10]

We pursued this observation when we conducted a randomized trial in Denmark, testing the potential beneficial nonspecific effects of neonatal BCG versus no BCG on morbidity. We asked whether the mother had been BCG vaccinated, hypothesizing that BCG would be particularly beneficial in children of BCG-vaccinated mothers. This turned out to be the case. Across all children in the trial, independently of their mothers' BCG status, neonatal BCG vaccination was not associated with a reduction in hospital admissions for infectious diseases.[11] However, consistent with our hypothesis, in the subgroup of children of BCG-vaccinated mothers (17% of participating children), randomization to BCG was associated with a 35% (95% CI: 6%–55%) lower rate of hospital admissions for infectious diseases, an effect that was significantly different from the effect observed in children of BCG-unvaccinated mothers.[11] BCG had also stronger beneficial effects in children of BCG-vaccinated mothers with respect to parental reports of infections (38% (95% CI: 2%–61% lower rate)) and general practitioner (GP) visits for infections (20% (95% CI: −3% to 38% lower rate) from 0 to 3 months of age,[12] and on atopic dermatitis up to 13 months of age (23% (95% CI: −1% to 42%) lower rate)).[13]

We subsequently explored whether this observation could be confirmed in Guinea-Bissau. After a correctly administered intradermal BCG vaccination, children normally develop a papule at the vaccination site that ulcerates and heals spontaneously, leaving a permanent scar. However, in studies from Guinea-Bissau, scar prevalence has been 52%–93%.[14,15] One may speculate that there are underlying immunological differences between children who develop and do not develop a scar. However, first, that would not explain the very varying scarification rate within a small and homogeneous population like the Guinean; second, we have found in both Guinea-Bissau and Denmark that the main reason for a lack of scar is incorrectly applied vaccination.[16,17] Thus, among BCG-vaccinated children, having a BCG scar can be interpreted as having had a correctly administered vaccination. This allows for an assessment of the effects of BCG vaccine among children who are otherwise similar in the sense that they were all presented for BCG vaccination at a health center (thus preventing confounding by a potential "healthy vaccinee effect"). We have found in several studies, comparing BCG scar versus no scar among BCG-vaccinated children, that a BCG scar is associated with strong mortality reductions.[14–16,18,19]

Within a randomized trial of early measles vaccine in Guinea-Bissau, we examined whether the mother and the child had a BCG scar at the time of enrolment at 4.5 months of age; the children were subsequently followed for mortality until 36 months of age.[20] We used that dataset to test the hypothesis that maternal BCG scarring enhanced the beneficial effects of having a BCG scar on offspring survival. For the 6227 children enrolled, 45% of the mothers and 86% of the children had a BCG scar. Children whose mother had a BCG scar were not more likely to have a BCG scar than children whose mother did not have a BCG scar (risk ratio 1.01 (95% CI: 0.99–1.03)).

In the main analysis, children who had a BCG scar had 41% (95% CI: 5%–64%) lower mortality between 4.5 and 36 months than children without a BCG scar. The reduction in mortality was 66% (95% CI: 33%–83%) if the mother had a BCG scar but only 8% (95% CI: −83% to 53%) if the mother had no BCG scar (test of interaction, $P = 0.04$) (submitted).

In conclusion, BCG had a particularly beneficial effect on morbidity and mortality in children whose mothers were BCG vaccinated, in Denmark[11–13] as well as in Guinea-Bissau (submitted). Hence, maternal priming with BCG may be important to elicit the beneficial nonspecific effects of BCG on morbidity and mortality. Whether paternal priming is important remains to be studied, but there is indeed increasing evidence of epigenetic inheritance through the male germ line,[21] which might play a role also for immune responses.

REVACCINATION WITH BCG ("BOOSTING")

Revaccination ("boosting") with BCG has also been associated with amplification of its beneficial nonspecific effects on mortality; the same has been seen for other live vaccines.[22] Two studies have examined BCG revaccination in relation to child survival.[23,24]

A large trial of 40,000 children was conducted in Algiers from 1935 to 1947, randomly allocating children to BCG or nothing at birth.[23] Three oral doses of BCG were provided with intervals of 2 days shortly after birth; the children were subsequently revaccinated at 1, 3, 7, and 11 years of age. The study provided no information on specific protection against TB or the proportion of deaths due to TB, but only on overall mortality. During the first year of life, the mortality in the BCG group was 3% (95% CI: −2% to 7%) lower than in the control group. A potential explanation might be that the initial doses provided at home by community nurses were often delayed, and because the analysis was intention-to-treat, deaths in the BCG group, which occurred prior to BCG vaccination, were included. After the first revaccination, overall child mortality was reduced by 17% (95% CI: 11%–22%) in the BCG group compared with the control group. After the second revaccination at 3 years, the reduction in mortality was 47% (95% CI: 38%–54%) between 3 and 4 years of age, a significant increase in effect (interaction tests, $P < 0.001$). Because follow-up visits were the same for the BCG-vaccinated and BCG-unvaccinated children, and because TB is unlikely to have caused many deaths in this young age group, the results indicated that BCG revaccination may have conferred strong additional beneficial nonspecific effects on child mortality.

More recently, we conducted a BCG revaccination trial in Guinea-Bissau. In Guinea-Bissau, nearly all children receive BCG early in life. Children were randomized to BCG revaccination or no vaccination at 19 months of age.[24] Among children, who had received the recommended diphtheria-tetanus-pertussis (DTP) booster vaccine at 18 months of age, before enrolment, and therefore did not get DTP booster after enrolment, BCG revaccination versus no BCG revaccination at 19 months of age was associated with a 64% (95% CI: 1%–87%) reduction in mortality between 19 months and 60 months of age.[24] However, if DTP booster was delivered after BCG, there was no beneficial effect of BCG revaccination; presumably DTP neutralized the beneficial effects of BCG revaccination.[24]

COMPARISON WITH OTHER VACCINES

As recently reviewed, all live attenuated vaccines for which there is data available, namely BCG, measles vaccine, smallpox vaccine, and oral polio vaccine, have been associated with beneficial nonspecific effects, and revaccination with these vaccines have been associated with additional benefits for child survival, which cannot be explained by the often very limited effect on overall mortality due to the target diseases.[22]

With respect to the potential effect on the beneficial nonspecific effects of vaccination in the presence of maternal immunity, so far only measles vaccine and BCG vaccines have been studied; for both vaccines, it seems particularly beneficial to be vaccinated in the presence of maternal immunity. For the two other live vaccines, smallpox vaccine and oral polio vaccine, it is unknown whether maternal priming leads to more beneficial effects of these vaccines on overall morbidity and mortality. It is difficult to study as smallpox vaccine was stopped since 1980, and oral polio vaccine is soon to be phased out.

Taken together, the data on BCG is backed by data on other live vaccines: additional doses, that is, doses given in the presence of existing immunity, from a previous vaccination or from the mother, confer additional nonspecific benefits on morbidity and mortality.

Interestingly, the effects of BCG immunotherapy against bladder cancer are stronger and more beneficial in patients who had received BCG vaccination prior to treatment initiation.[25]

IMMUNOLOGICAL MECHANISMS

It is well known that maternal antibody can dampen the specific antibody responses to a vaccine, whereas it does not hamper T-cell priming.[9] The two immune mechanisms mediating the influence of maternal antibody on infant vaccine responses seem to be specific masking of B-cell determinants and antigen-presenting cell uptake of maternal antibody-antigen complexes, which are readily internalized, and can lead to a more enhanced T-cell over B-cell response.[9,10] Whether other forms of maternal immunity than antibodies influence child immune responses to vaccines is unknown.

With respect to maternal priming with BCG, it was recently shown infants of mothers with a BCG scar, compared with infants of mothers without a BCG scar, had overall higher proinflammatory cytokine responses 1 and 6 weeks following neonatal BCG vaccination; the expression of genes in the interferon and inflammation responses pathways was also increased.[26] The study did not include BCG-unvaccinated neonates but does indicate that maternal BCG vaccination may have a profound impact on the offspring.

With respect to BCG revaccination, a human study has shown that BCG vaccination induced an antibody response, which was enhanced after a revaccination with BCG 6 months later. It was proposed that this was because preexisting antibodies enhanced the internalization of BCG by neutrophils and monocytes.[27] In mice, preopsonization of BCG with anti-BCG-IgG potentiated phagocytosis by macrophages, and led to increased nitric oxide (NO) production.[28] BCG has been shown to induce epigenetic modifications of monocytes via stimulation of the intracellular NOD2-receptor, which lead to increased innate immune responses upon a secondary encounter of (unrelated) pathogens, so-called "trained innate immunity".[6] This effect is still partially present after a year, but may wane over time.[29]

Thus, the beneficial effect of BCG vaccination in the presence of preexisting immunity may represent increased internalization of BCG by monocytes, increased NOD2 activation, and NO production, mediating stronger epigenetic effects leading to enhanced trained innate immunity.

Whether the enhancing effect of pre-existing immunity is caused by vaccine-induced antibodies or cellular immunity, for example, by epigenetic modifications is not clear. Both humoral factors (antibodies) and epigenetic imprinting may be transferred transgenerationally,[9,30] hence in fact both mechanisms may be in play.

CONCLUSION AND PERSPECTIVES

The present data on BCG suggests that we may be designed to benefit from meeting BCG in the presence of preexisting immunity, be it from our mother or from previous exposure, and we may benefit from continued exposure.[22] If this is correct, there are a number of potential implications. First, we should ensure that girls (and maybe boys) are BCG-vaccinated (i.e., have a BCG scar) before they become parents. Second, we should strive to provide BCG to the child as early as possible; currently, BCG at birth is a policy in TB-endemic countries, but BCG is often given with delay, implicating waning of the maternally inherited immunity. Third, we should revaccinate all children who do not develop a BCG scar after the first vaccination. Fourth, we should probably revaccinate all children with BCG once or more during childhood. Fifth, we should make sure that all bladder cancer patients due to receive BCG bladder installments are given an intradermal BCG prior to treatment. Most of this would, of course, require further studies, but the potential gains indicated by the existing evidence suggest that such studies are urgently warranted.

REFERENCES

1. Biering-Sørensen S, Aaby P, Lund N, Monteiro I, Jensen KJ, Eriksen HB, et al. Early BCG-Denmark and neonatal mortality among infants weighing <2500 g: a randomized controlled trial. *Clin Inf Dis*. 2017;65(7):1183–1190.
2. Higgins JP, Soares-Weiser K, Lopez-Lopez JA, Kakourou A, Chaplin K, Christensen H, et al. Association of BCG, DTP, and measles containing vaccines with childhood mortality: systematic review. *BMJ*. 2016;355:i5170.
3. Aaby P, Kollmann TR, Benn CS. Nonspecific effects of neonatal and infant vaccination: public-health, immunological and conceptual challenges. *Nat Immunol*. 2014;15(10):895–899.
4. Rieckmann A, Villumsen M, Sorup S, Haugaard LK, Ravn H, Roth A, et al. Vaccinations against smallpox and tuberculosis are associated with better long-term survival: a Danish case-cohort study 1971–2010. *Int J Epidemiol*. 2017;46(2):695–705.
5. Benn CS, Netea MG, Selin LK, Aaby P. A small jab—a big effect: nonspecific immunomodulation by vaccines. *Trends Immunol*. 2013;34(9):431–439.
6. Kleinnijenhuis J, Quintin J, Preijers F, Joosten LA, Ifrim DC, Saeed S, et al. Bacille Calmette-Guerin induces NOD2-dependent nonspecific protection from reinfection via epigenetic reprogramming of monocytes. *Proc Natl Acad Sci U S A*. 2012;109(43):17537–17542.
7. Aaby P, Benn CS. Saving lives by training innate immunity with bacille Calmette-Guerin vaccine. *Proc Natl Acad Sci U S A*. 2012;109(43):17317–17318.
8. Blok BA, Arts RJ, van Crevel R, Benn CS, Netea MG. Trained innate immunity as underlying mechanism for the long-term, nonspecific effects of vaccines. *J Leuk Biol*. 2015;98(3):347–356.
9. Siegrist CA. Mechanisms by which maternal antibodies influence infant vaccine responses: review of hypotheses and definition of main determinants. *Vaccine*. 2003;21(24):3406–3412.
10. Aaby P, Martins CL, Garly ML, Andersen A, Fisker AB, Claesson MH, et al. Measles vaccination in the presence or absence of maternal measles antibody: impact on child survival. *Clin Infect Dis*. 2014;59(4):484–492.
11. Stensballe LG, Ravn H, Birk NM, Kjærgaard J, Nissen TN, Pihl GT, et al. BCG vaccination at birth and rate of hospitalization for infection until 15 months of age in Danish children: a randomized clinical multicenter trial. *J Pediatric Infect Dis Soc*. 2018. https://doi.org/10.1093/jpids/piy029.
12. Kjaergaard J, Birk NM, Nissen TN, Thostesen LM, Pihl GT, Benn CS, et al. Nonspecific effect of BCG vaccination at birth on early childhood infections: a randomized, clinical multicenter trial. *Pediatr Res*. 2016;80(5):681–685.
13. Thostesen LM, Kjaergaard J, Pihl GT, Birk NM, Nissen TN, Aaby P, et al. Neonatal BCG vaccination and atopic dermatitis before 13 months of age: a randomized clinical trial. *Allergy*. 2017;.
14. Storgaard L, Rodrigues A, Martins C, Nielsen BU, Ravn H, Benn CS, et al. Development of BCG scar and subsequent morbidity and mortality in rural Guinea-Bissau. *Clin Infect Dis*. 2015;61(6):950–959.

15. Timmermann CA, Biering-Sorensen S, Aaby P, Fisker AB, Monteiro I, Rodrigues A, et al. Tuberculin reaction and BCG scar: association with infant mortality. *Trop Med Int Health*. 2015;20(12):1733–1744.
16. Roth A, Sodemann M, Jensen H, Poulsen A, Gustafson P, Weise C, et al. Tuberculin reaction, BCG scar, and lower female mortality. *Epidemiology*. 2006;17(5):562–568.
17. Birk NM, Nissen TN, Ladekarl M, Zingmark V, Kjaergaard J, Jensen TM, et al. The association between Bacillus Calmette-Guerin vaccination (1331 SSI) skin reaction and subsequent scar development in infants. *BMC Infect Dis*. 2017;17(1):540.
18. Garly ML, Martins CL, Bale C, Balde MA, Hedegaard KL, Gustafson P, et al. BCG scar and positive tuberculin reaction associated with reduced child mortality in West Africa. A non-specific beneficial effect of BCG? *Vaccine*. 2003;21(21–22):2782–2790.
19. Roth A, Gustafson P, Nhaga A, Djana Q, Poulsen A, Garly ML, et al. BCG vaccination scar associated with better childhood survival in Guinea-Bissau. *Int J Epidemiol*. 2005;34(3):540–547.
20. Aaby P, Martins CL, Garly ML, Bale C, Andersen A, Rodrigues A, et al. Non-specific effects of standard measles vaccine at 4.5 and 9 months of age on childhood mortality: randomised controlled trial. *BMJ*. 2010;341:c6495.
21. Soubry A, Hoyo C, Jirtle RL, Murphy SK. A paternal environmental legacy: evidence for epigenetic inheritance through the male germ line. *Bioessays*. 2014;36(4):359–371.
22. Benn CS, Fisker AB, Whittle HC, Aaby P. Revaccination with live attenuated vaccines confer additional beneficial nonspecific effects on overall survival: a review. *EBioMedicine*. 2016;10:312–317.
23. Sergent E. Premunition antituberculose par le BCG. Campagne poursuive depuis 1935 sur 21,244 nouveau-nes vaccines et 20,063 non vaccines: premiere note. *Arch Inst Pastuer Alger*. 1954;32(1):1–8.
24. Roth AE, Benn CS, Ravn H, Rodrigues A, Lisse IM, Yazdanbakhsh M, et al. Effect of revaccination with BCG in early childhood on mortality: randomised trial in Guinea-Bissau. *BMJ*. 2010;340:c671.
25. Biot C, Rentsch CA, Gsponer JR, Birkhauser FD, Jusforgues-Saklani H, Lemaitre F, et al. Preexisting BCG-specific T cells improve intravesical immunotherapy for bladder cancer. *Sci Transl Med*. 2012;4(137):137ra72.
26. Mawa PA, Webb EL, Filali-Mouhim A, Nkurunungi G, Sekaly RP, Lule SA, et al. Maternal BCG scar is associated with increased infant proinflammatory immune responses. *Vaccine*. 2017;35(2):273–282.
27. de Valliere S, Abate G, Blazevic A, Heuertz RM, Hoft DF. Enhancement of innate and cell-mediated immunity by antimycobacterial antibodies. *Infect Immun*. 2005;73(10):6711–6720.
28. Silva MC, Lasunskaia EB, Silva WD. Repeated inoculations of Mycobacterium bovis Bacille Calmette-Guerin (BCG) are needed to induce a strong humoral immune response against antigens expressed by the bacteria. *Open J Immunol*. 2013;03(03):71–81.
29. Kleinnijenhuis J, Quintin J, Preijers F, Benn CS, Joosten LA, Jacobs C, et al. Long-lasting effects of BCG vaccination on both heterologous Th1/Th17 responses and innate trained immunity. *J Innate Immun*. 2014;6(2):152–158.
30. Prokopuk L, Western PS, Stringer JM. Transgenerational epigenetic inheritance: adaptation through the germline epigenome? *Epigenomics*. 2015;7(5):829–846.

INDEX

Note: Page numbers followed by *f* indicate figures, and *t* indicate tables.